MINDFUL EATING

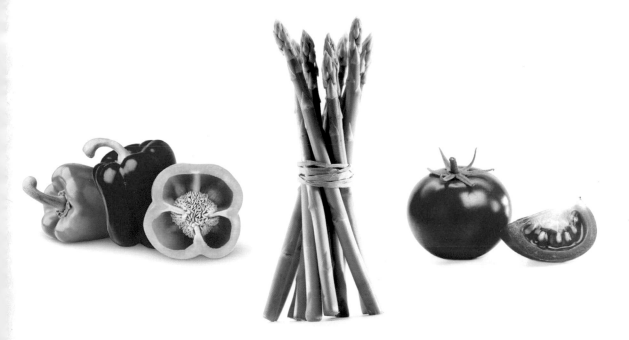

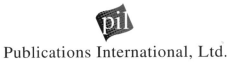

Publications International, Ltd.

Publications International, Ltd.

Table of Contents

MINDFUL EATING

WHAT IS MINDFULNESS?

Imagine you are sitting in a car, on your usual morning commute. The radio is on, traffic is bad, and you're thinking about the day ahead. Maybe you have a deadline to meet or an important project to work on. Your mind wanders, you grip the steering wheel tightly, and then you absentmindedly reach for your coffee in the cup-holder, gulping some down while watching the brake lights of the car in front of you. By the time you arrive at work, your mind is a swirling jumble of thoughts. You barely even remember the drive from your house. And you certainly don't remember drinking all that coffee.

Now, what if you tried something different on your morning commute? The next day, as you're in your car, sitting in traffic, you switch off the radio. You listen to the silence, or the sound of the car engine, or the sound

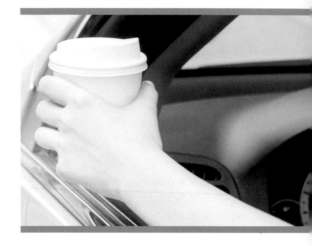

of your own breathing. You take a deep breath and inhale the heavenly aroma of coffee from the mug in the cup-holder. You pay attention to your own body language, you make note of the colors of the cars around you, and you pay attention to the landmarks you pass. Instead of gulping down your coffee, you pick up the mug and take a small sip. You notice the temperature of the hot beverage and savor the taste. Instead of allowing your mind to fill up with to-dos and worries, you simply focus on the present.

You've just had a moment of mindfulness.

In the simplest sense, "mindfulness" is paying attention to thoughts, feelings, and surroundings as they occur. In other words, mindfulness is being present in the present. It seems like it should be easy—after all, the only place we can actually live is in the present. The past is gone, never to return, and the future is unknown and uncertain, yet we allow thoughts of the past and worry about the future to consume our lives. But why? Since we don't live in the past or future, all of this regret, worry and speculation can be unproductive and cause us undo stress. Making a conscious effort to focus on the present is one way to help alleviate some of this stress. Mindfulness can be a tool to help us live more fulfilled and less anxious lives.

Although it sounds a bit like a trendy buzzword, the practice of mindfulness has been around for millennia. The word "mindfulness" was derived from the word "sati" from the Pali language. Pali is the sacred language of Buddhism, where sati, what we call mindfulness, is considered one of the "Seven Factors of Enlightenment." Other Eastern religions, such as Hinduism and Taoism, also embraced the idea of mindfulness long before it made its way to the Western world even as early as 1500 B.C.

By contrast, the practice didn't begin to take hold in Western psychology until the late 1970s. In 1979, a professor at the University of Massachusetts, Jon Kabat-Zinn, created a program called mindfulness-based stress reduction, or MBSR. Kabat-Zinn had studied yoga and meditation with Buddhist teachers and was one of the founding members of the Cambridge Zen Center in Cambridge, Massachusetts. He became fascinated by the idea of combining his Buddhist teachings with science-based approaches to reducing stress, anxiety, and worry. His MBSR program made use of mindfulness methods to help people cope with negative feelings. The program, which consists of an eight-week-long workshop complete with 45 minutes of daily "homework," became so popular that today it is used by hospitals, schools, businesses, and prisons as a way to help people reduce stress and control emotions.

Fortunately, you don't have to attend a long workshop, be a Buddhist monk, or even go to a yoga class to make use of mindfulness. Anyone can use the ideas found in the philosophy, anytime. There are several tenets that define the concept of mindfulness, and understanding them is the first step to a calmer mind and a healthier lifestyle.

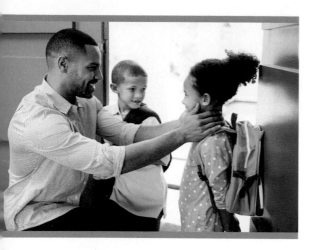

FOCUS ON THE PRESENT MOMENT

The main goal of mindfulness is, of course, to focus on the present moment. It can take some effort to resist the temptation of wistfully recalling past situations or fretting about what the future may hold, but like anything else, mindfulness gets easier the more you practice.

There are two ways that you can focus on your present moment. One is through "concentrated" mindfulness, when you focus on one single item or thought at a time, even if it seems inconsequential. "Diffuse" mindfulness, on the other hand, is taking note of your entire surroundings, and paying attention to the thoughts and feelings you have at a single moment.

Mindfulness can also be categorized as formal or informal. Formal mindfulness is simply meditation. It can take a bit of planning to find a quiet location where you won't be interrupted, but formal mindfulness can be quite useful to instill a sense of peace and calm.

Since it's not always practical to find moments of solitude and quiet, many of us don't make use of mediation in our daily lives. When it's difficult to steal away to a quiet location, informal mindfulness can come in handy. Informal mindfulness is having a present awareness of your day-to-day life, no matter what you're doing. You could be driving the kids to school, giving a presentation, or cooking dinner, and still find a way to be mindful. You can pay attention to details and feelings throughout the day, living in each moment.

WILLINGNESS TO ACCEPT EXPERIENCES

Another tenet of mindfulness is the willingness to accept all experiences, including negative experiences. This can be difficult, because we often attempt to avoid negative feelings out of fear. Although it may seem counterintuitive, when we are mindful, we don't shut out these negative emotions. Rather, we actually allow them to occur, and accept the fact that these things are a part of life. Mindfulness teaches us that not only should we accept our negative thoughts and feelings, but also that it is okay to have negative thoughts and feelings. At that point those emotions lose their power over us, and what's more, we are able to understand that we have power over them.

VIEWING FEELINGS IN A NON-JUDGMENTAL WAY

Another important philosophy when practicing mindfulness is perceiving emotions and experiences without judgment. This means that negative emotions should not be considered "bad," and positive emotions should not be considered "good." Rather, when being mindful, emotions are simply accepted. And our reactions to positive or negative emotions should be the same.

ACCEPTANCE OF PRESENT REALITY

Inventor Alexander Graham Bell once said, "When one door closes another door opens; but we so often look so long and so regretfully upon the closed door, that we do not see the ones which open for us." Who hasn't looked into the past and wished they could reopen a closed door? Most people are guilty of gazing too long at one of those closed doors, and we probably miss out on new opportunities because of it.

And longing for the past isn't our only mistake—we also worry about the future. But when so much of our future is uncertain, why do we spend such a disproportionally large amount of time obsessing over it? Mindfulness teaches that instead of longing for the past or worrying about the future, we should focus on the present and accept our existing situation.

NON-ATTACHMENT

Now, don't misunderstand—accepting the present doesn't mean we have to be resigned to live in a stagnant situation for the rest of our lives. Just because we focus on and accept the present doesn't mean we must remain mired in motionless inaction. On the

> *"The best way to capture moments is to pay attention. This is how we cultivate mindfulness. Mindfulness means being awake. It means knowing what you are doing."*
>
> *~Jon Kabat-Zinn*

contrary, mindfulness recognizes that life is in a constant state of change. Because of that, it is important to look at our situations with a sense of non-attachment; this makes the idea of change easier to handle.

PATIENCE, PEACE, AND TRUST

Finally, approach the practice of mindfulness with an attitude of patience, peace, and trust. Although your mind may wander at first, with practice, it will be easier to be mindful and maintain focus on the present. Have patience, also, with whatever changes you hope to see. Whether it be a better attitude, a healthier lifestyle or more motivation, changes don't always appear overnight.

As many of the other tenets suggest, it is also important to practice mindfulness with a sense of peace. After all, it can be difficult to be non-judgmental toward negative feelings if you don't first approach them with a peaceful attitude. Always strive to maintain an even keel, no matter what is happening in your present situation. Things won't always work out the way you hoped, but a peaceful acceptance of the moment will make it easier to continue moving forward.

And trust in your own intuition and feelings while you practice mindfulness. Trust that the changes you are hoping for will occur, in their own time. And trust that you have all the strength and tools that you need within you to live a healthier, more balanced lifestyle.

DOES MINDFULNESS REALLY WORK?

The short answer is: yes! And now that you have a better understanding of the ideas that form the basis for mindfulness, you can try out the practice for yourself.

The ancient practitioners of mindfulness believed it to be a way to promote well being and peace, and it turns out that modern science supports this assumption. When Kabat-Zinn first created his MBSR program, one of the discoveries he made was that the practice of mindfulness helped to alleviate chronic pain in patients with debilitating illnesses. Scientists exploring the practice noticed that when patients focused on the present and used the tools they learned in the MBSR program, certain areas of their brains were more active, including a part of the brain responsible for resilience. This means that when we practice mindfulness, we become more willing to tackle problems head-on, as opposed to hiding from them or running away.

Resilience isn't the only improved function researchers have found. After using MRI machines to scan the brains of people before and after mindfulness sessions, scientists discovered that people who embrace mindfulness are also more likely to embrace their experiences and less likely to criticize themselves. Another thing researchers have found is that the "fight or flight" area of the brain actually shrinks after practicing mindfulness, meaning that the body is less likely to have a severe response to stress. So even when life gets hectic, crazy, or tense, you are better able to handle it. You feel less fear when dealing with a stressful situation and are able to recover from negativity more easily.

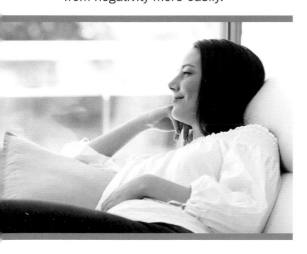

But perhaps the most amazing discovery scientists have made about mindfulness is that patients who regularly engage in mindful behavior actually improve their immune systems. And in addition to providing pain relief, helping to cope with difficult thoughts and situations, and instilling those who practice with feelings of self-acceptance, mindfulness practice has also been shown to lower blood pressure, decrease anxiety and depression, help with addictions, eating disorders, and obsessive-compulsive behavior, and improve focus and concentration. Mindfulness has even been shown to decrease drug use and increase optimism in prison inmates, and reduce the likelihood of a relapse of criminal behavior.

This is not to say that practicing mindfulness will cure diseases or solve every problem you have, but the science seems to agree that it can provide you with some concrete tools to live a healthier life.

MINDFULNESS IN OUR DAILY LIVES

FORMAL MINDFULNESS

Formal mindfulness, or mindfulness meditation, can be a great tool to help you prepare for a long day or unwind at night. To start, find a quiet location and a comfortable seat. You can sit in a chair, or just sit on the floor, if you prefer. Begin by focusing on your breathing—the steady "in" and "out" of each breath. If you like, you can focus on a single word, like "calm" or "peace" or any other word that resonates with you.

Now pay attention to the way your body feels, and observe any sights or sounds nearby. As you sit quietly, allow your thoughts to come and go, and take note of the emotions each thought conjures up. Remember to observe everything without judgement and to accept your thoughts as they occur.

Some experts believe that the most benefit from mindfulness meditation comes from 20 minutes of meditation a day. If that seems like a long time to sit quietly, start with just a few minutes, and work your way up to longer sessions. It may feel awkward at first to practice mindfulness meditation, but with some time and patience, you may find that it becomes an integral part of your daily routine.

THE INFORMAL OPTION

If meditation just isn't your thing, or your day is too busy to squeeze in some solitude, informal mindfulness is something anyone can fit into their schedule, anytime. For informal mindfulness, you don't necessarily need to be in a quiet location, although it may help to have fewer distractions as you get used to the process. The key is to remember to stay focused on the present, even when things get hectic.

One way to practice mindfulness throughout the day is by pausing before taking an action. So before you head into the office, take a few minutes to quietly sit at your desk or in your car before tackling the tasks of the day. Take a few deep breaths, take note of the sights and sounds nearby, and allow your thoughts and feelings to come and go. You can also pause in other areas of the day—before answering a ringing phone, for example, or before heading into a meeting. Simply take a quick deep breath, or pause to collect your thoughts, and focus on your feelings.

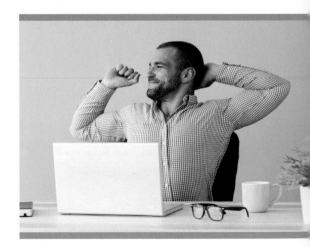

Continue practicing mindfulness in these ways throughout your work day and on your commute home, and perhaps you'll discover that you have a calmer, more productive day. Once at home, you can sneak in more moments of mindfulness in between family obligations or distractions. For instance, if you cook dinner, pay extra attention to the process. Take note of the texture of vegetables, and listen to the sound each makes when you chop and slice. And of course, be sure to inhale each aroma of the cooking process.

Once it's time to wind down for the evening, mindfulness can be a great tool to help you fall asleep. Start by removing distractions. Turn off the television and computer, and try to avoid your phone or tablet screens as well. These screens emit a short wavelength blue light, which mimics sunlight and tricks your brain into thinking it's still daytime. If your mind is racing with thoughts of the day, as tends to happen with our busy lives, just allow the thoughts to come and go. Spend some time focusing on how you feel, both physically and mentally. The beauty of informal mindfulness is that it really is about moment-to-moment awareness, whether those moments are chaotic and noisy ones during the day or more calm and relaxing ones in the evening.

MINDFULNESS AND MEALS

In the early 20th century, a self-proclaimed nutritionist and businessman by the name of Horace Fletcher proposed some interesting ideas about eating. Fletcher believed that during a meal, each bite of food should be thoroughly chewed—approximately 32 chews per bite, one bite for each tooth—before being swallowed. All of this chewing, he believed, would help to jump-start the digestion process and help the body absorb nutrients without absorbing as many calories. Fletcher also told his followers that they should eat only when hungry, and they should refrain from eating when feeling angry or sad. And, he said, they should pay attention to what sorts of ingredients were in their food, as different foods produced different "waste products," and obviously people needed to be aware of these details.

Chewing a bite of food dozens of times definitely seems like a bit of overkill. But it turns out that Fletcher may have been on to something. Studies have found that when people chew their food more, they end up eating up to 12 percent fewer calories overall. And it's hard to argue with the logic of only eating when hungry, or of being aware of what sorts of ingredients are in the foods we put into our bodies. These ideas may have seemed radical in the Victorian era, but nowadays they line right up with what nutritionists and dietitians preach. Fletcher was even on the right track when he advocated abstaining from eating when feeling emotional. In a way, Horace Fletcher may have been ahead of his time—he was, perhaps inadvertently, one of the first practitioners of mindful eating.

If you're like many people, chances are you don't always eat in a mindful way. Think about a typical day with typical mealtimes. Breakfast might be rushed as you hurry to get yourself and the rest of your household out the door. Maybe you grab a quick slice of toast before heading out. Or perhaps you eat something in your car during your commute, or swig some coffee, not really paying much attention to it. Lunch may be at your desk at work, where you don't necessarily take a real break. By the time you're home and ready for dinner, you're tired and hungry. Maybe you don't feel like cooking, so you just throw something in the microwave. Or perhaps you order out and have food delivered. Either way, you end up in front of the television, a plate on your lap, paying more attention to the screen than whatever you're putting in your mouth.

Many of us eat our meals in this way—we eat, but we don't really pay much attention to the process. We try to be great multi-taskers, so we combine mealtimes with other errands and responsibilities, like driving or reading emails or folding laundry. Even worse is when we "indulge" in some kind of "diet" food—food that has been made "better" or lower calorie by replacing fat and sugar with artificial ingredients. But these "better" foods are never as satisfying as the real deal. The result of all this mindless eating is, at best,

a lack of appreciation for the abundant food we have, and at worst, the possibility of weight gain and a sense of dissatisfaction with mealtimes. And if you're not satisfied after you eat, this often leads to more eating. It can be difficult to break the cycle, but that's where mindful eating can step in.

> *"In today's rush, we all think too much—seek too much—want too much—and forget about the joy of just being."*
>
> ~Eckhart Tolle, author and spiritual teacher

WHAT IS MINDFUL EATING?

When we practice mindfulness, we try to use all of our senses to observe the present moment. With mindful eating, we do the same. Instead of eating food without thought to what we're doing, we deliberately pay attention to each bite, taking note of the appearance, smell, texture, taste, and even sound of the food we eat. And just as we approach our emotions in a non-judgmental way when we practice mindfulness, we do the same with mindful eating—we try not to think of any particular food as "good" or "bad," and we taste foods without allowing our perception of them to alter our experience. This practice can help us develop a healthier relationship to our food.

In their book *The Mindful Way through Depression: Freeing Yourself from Chronic Unhappiness,* authors Mark Williams, John Teasdale, Zindel Segal, and Jon Kabat-Zinn use the example of eating one single raisin to describe the nuances of mindful eating. Through an eight-step process, they describe how we can practice mindful eating even with the tiniest bites of food. So grab a raisin—or, if you don't have any raisins in your pantry, feel free to use a grape, a single corn flake, a chocolate chip, or any other small bite of food—and try out a quick mindful eating exercise:

The first step is to hold the raisin (or whichever food you've chosen). Place it between your thumb and finger as you move on to step two: See it. Look at the raisin and pay attention to what you see. Take note of the curves and ridges of the fruit. Now spend a few moments observing the texture, turning the raisin over in your fingers and using your sense of touch. Next, engage your sense of smell: Hold the raisin to your nose and inhale the fragrance.

Now it's time to place the raisin in your mouth, but don't chew it yet. Just observe the sensation of the food in your mouth and the way it feels on your

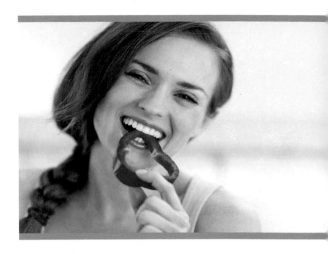

tongue. Next, begin to chew slowly, taking note of where the raisin is in your mouth and what the first taste is like. Notice how the texture changes as you chew. When you feel like you're ready, swallow the raisin. And finally, follow up the whole exercise by observing anything you feel afterwards.

Eating mindfully in this way can help us to enjoy our food more, which can actually help us to feel satisfied even when we eat less. One of the things that makes our eating experiences a bit more complicated is the hormone that regulates fullness. The intestinal tract secretes a hormone called ghrelin to signal your brain that it's time to stop eating. Experts have noted that it takes about 20 minutes for the ghrelin signal to reach the brain and cause you to feel full. When we eat quickly or without paying attention, we risk overeating before we even realize we're full. We end up with that uncomfortable bloated feeling, and probably a mind full of regret.

Not only that, but when we eat mindlessly, our food is much less enjoyable. Food tastes good, and if we eat too quickly or with distractions, we're less likely to notice even the most delicious tastes. Mindful eating can help us to not only fuel our bodies with the nutrients it needs, but to also enjoy the experience!

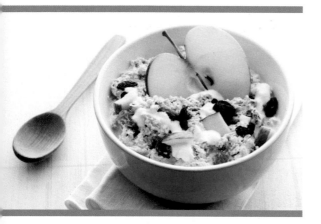

PRINCIPLES OF MINDFUL EATING

SLOW DOWN

One of the most basic ideas—and perhaps most important—is to slow down. Many times we eat quickly, without even thinking about it. Mindful eating requires a slower pace—you need time to pay attention to what you're eating, so you can engage your senses and savor the experience. You may not always have the time to

devote to mindful eating, and that's okay. Sometimes mornings are rushed and work is busy, and it's not always practical to sit down and eat slowly. But try to set aside at least one or two meals a week for mindful eating, and you may find that you enjoy it so much, you strive to do it more often.

LOSE THE DISTRACTIONS

You should also try to eat without distractions. In other words, don't multitask while you're eating. Try not to eat in the car, step away from the computer during lunch, and turn off the television before dinner. You can turn off your phone or leave it in another room so you're not tempted to scroll through social media while you eat. This makes it easier to pay attention, not only to what your food smells and tastes like, but to how you feel as you're eating. You'll be better able to recognize when you're full if you're not distracted by work or noise.

PAY ATTENTION TO HUNGER CUES

Another principle of mindful eating is using hunger cues to dictate when you should eat. Eating when we're not hungry seems to be another byproduct of our convenient society—since food is constantly available, we don't think twice about eating, whether or not we want or need to. This is not to say that you should wait to eat until you're starving—this can be its own danger, because ravenous hunger can lead to crankiness and poor decisions. Instead of making a healthy choice to eat, you're more likely to reach for some convenient junk food and devour it before you have time to consider whether it's the best thing for your body. With mindful eating, the key is to pay close attention to your own body's hunger cues. Remember that mindfulness teaches us to pause before we act. Pause before you reach for a snack, and ask yourself whether you really need it. Sometimes the answer will be yes, and that's okay, but many times you'll discover that your desire for food is simply stemming from boredom or stress.

DON'T JUDGE

Mindfulness teaches us that there are no "bad" or "good" feelings, and the same idea applies to mindful eating. When we eat mindfully, there is no such thing as "good" food or "bad" food. Rather, with mindful eating, we attempt to recognize the foods that will nourish us, while also appreciating the foods that simply taste good. When all food is given an even plane, none of it seems forbidden or more virtuous than any other. It becomes easier to eat a healthy diet, while also realizing that treats and special indulgences aren't off-limits. In fact, in our attempt to make foods that we've

deemed "bad" into "good" foods, we've really sabotaged ourselves. Supermarket aisles are lined with low-fat and low-calorie cookies and ice cream, the results of our desire to be "better" about what we eat. But if you had the choice between two or three low-fat cookies made with a few unpronounceable ingredients or one regular cookie made with butter and chocolate and vanilla, chances are you'd want the one regular cookie because it would be much more satisfying. So when we buy those low-fat cookies, with the intention to eat "better," we may end up eating even more than we would if we simply stuck to good old-fashioned cookies, because one of the "better" cookies isn't nearly as satisfying.

And once again, just as with mindfulness, we practice non-judgment when eating mindfully. This means that when you take a bite of food and decide you hate it, you accept your reaction without judgment. Likewise, when you love a food, you simply acknowledge the feeling and move on.

USE YOUR SENSES

Lastly, when we eat mindfully, we use all of our senses. Think back to the single raisin example: You not only tasted the raisin, but you looked at it, touched it, and smelled it, as well. You can even engage your sense of hearing with some foods—crunchy carrots, for example, or the light crackle of the caramelized sugar on a crème brûlée. The point is to just pay attention to the entire experience when you eat, instead of mindlessly putting food in your mouth. You may discover that there is so much more to enjoy about eating than simply the taste of your food.

BENEFITS OF MINDFUL EATING

LESS FOOD, MORE SATISFACTION

Start with the first principle—slowing down. In the late 1980s, researchers noticed that even though the French diet was high in foods like cheese, butter and pastries, the French people had a lower risk of obesity. Even today, obesity rates in France are about half of what they are in the United States. Yet French croissants are famous for their copious amounts of butter, and French wine is coveted by many a sommelier. So how can the French eat cheese and croissants and not struggle with the obesity rates of the U.S.?

Part of the answer may lie in how the French approach mealtimes. In France, lunch at a restaurant can stretch on for two hours. People take the time to enjoy their food, by savoring one bite at a time before moving on to another. Eating in this way can actually make our food taste better as well. Have you ever noticed that your first bite of

chocolate cake tastes much better than the last? This is because our taste buds "tire out" after tasting the same thing over and over. But if we pause for a few moments before taking another bite, our sense of taste is sharper, and we enjoy the food more.

Another way the French get it right is by serving smaller portions. Sure, they eat cheese and pastries, but they eat less of them. And remember, it takes about 20 minutes for your body to tell your brain that you're full. By slowing down, focusing on each bite, and taking the time your body needs to process the meal, it takes less food to feel more satisfied. You can eat a smaller portion and still feel like you had plenty to eat. So not only does eating slowly help you to enjoy each bite of food more, but it ensures that you'll recognize your satiety signals before you become uncomfortably full.

As we've talked about, it's also important to rid yourself of distractions when practicing mindful eating. Researchers are discovering that eating without distractions may be even more important than anyone realized. When we eat in a distracted manner, our brains may only record the other things we are doing—driving or replying to emails, for instance—and we forget that we ate anything at all. Once again, we eat an entire meal, but end up feeling unsatisfied because the experience hasn't been stored in our memory. Even more troubling, there is evidence that eating while distracted actually slows the digestion process. We're left with another negative cycle: We eat while we're distracted, which leaves us unsatisfied. So we eat more, even though our digestive system is still working on our previous meal!

UNDERSTANDING YOUR HUNGER

Another principle of mindful eating is paying attention to hunger cues. This isn't always as simple as "I'm hungry" or "I'm not hungry." Emotional eating is a genuine problem—who hasn't turned to food during times of stress, exhaustion or boredom? While it's not always a bad thing to simply eat for the sake of eating (perhaps at a party or special occasion), when it becomes a habit, it can be a problem. You begin to associate your feelings with food, and eating for emotional reasons creates an unhealthy cycle.

Emotional hunger and physical hunger are not the same thing, and mindful eating can help you sort through the differences. Physical hunger comes on gradually and doesn't feel as urgent as emotional hunger. With emotional hunger, the feeling hits you suddenly, and it can seem like you have to eat something right at that moment. And the food you crave when you eat for emotional reasons is usually a comfort food—the idea of vegetables or grilled chicken might sound great when

you're physically hungry, but emotional hunger usually demands sugary, fatty, or salty foods.

Emotional hunger often goes hand in hand with mindless eating. When you're stressed or upset, you're less likely to pay attention to what you're eating. You just dig in to a pint of ice cream and can hardly remember where it went once it's gone. And then, even though you've eaten more than enough calories, you're not satisfied. With physical hunger, you feel satisfied after you've eaten, if you don't feel stuffed. But emotional hunger is different—it doesn't matter how much you eat, you're still unsatisfied afterwards.

What's more, emotional hunger obviously doesn't originate in your stomach, where physical hunger begins. When you're physically hungry, you can feel stomach pangs or an emptiness in your belly that tells you it's time to eat. But emotional hunger starts in your mind. The craving you feel isn't physical, it's mental, and often leaves you feeling guilty or ashamed.

Mindful eating can help you to gain control over emotional hunger. One of the tools we can use when practicing mindfulness is to pause before acting, which can be especially useful when it comes to sorting out the differences between your physical hunger and emotional hunger. Before you eat something, take a few moments to think about why you want to eat at that moment. Are you feeling actual physical hunger cues or are they emotional cues? Emotional eating tends to have triggers, so think about whether something is triggering your desire to eat. Are you feeling stress about a situation in your life? What about your emotional state: Are you feeling sad, angry, anxious, or afraid? Maybe you're just bored, or you've conditioned yourself to eat something out of habit. If any of these sound familiar, chances are you're eating because of emotional hunger.

Identifying emotional hunger by mindfully considering your food choices is the first step to conquering emotional eating. Once you've done that, you can focus on finding other ways to cope with your feelings. If you're feeling stressed, find a way to take care of yourself: Do something you love, like read a book or watch a favorite movie. If you're feeling depressed or lonely, call a friend, find something funny to watch on television, or write in a journal. Exercise is always a great choice, as well, since working out is proven to reduce anxiety and depression. And even if you still end up eating something after you've paused to consider your reasons, you'll have a better understanding of why you did it.

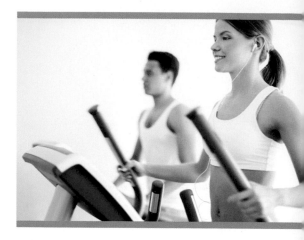

The principle of non-judgment can also come in handy when we are identifying hunger cues. As mindfulness teaches us, we should acknowledge and accept our feelings without judging them; these feelings are neither good nor bad. And when we accept our feelings, we can recognize that there are other ways to handle them besides eating. We don't necessarily have to eat when we feel emotional hunger; we can just acknowledge the cravings we have and move forward.

LOSING THE LABELS

Non-judgement applies to more than just our feelings. It applies to the food we eat as well. When we stop labeling food as "good" or "bad," it loses some of its power over us, just as our emotions lose power over us when we stop thinking of them in positive and negative terms. If you're always thinking about chocolate cake as a "bad" food that you shouldn't eat, then when you eat a slice, you might end up feeling guilty about it afterwards. And you may feel good about yourself after you eat a salad, but subconsciously, that virtuous feeling may lead you to eat more of your "bad" foods later on.

This is just one of the ways we sabotage ourselves when we start putting labels on different foods. With mindful eating, we pay attention to the nuances of our food, but we do so without judgement. Think back to the French example: We may consider cheese and croissants "bad" food, yet the people of France continue to eat them without shame. And perhaps this is because to them, cheese and croissants are simply "food." Food to be enjoyed, one bite at a time.

Of course, the main purpose of eating food is to nourish and fuel our bodies, so obviously we can't spend all our time eating cake and croissants. Even though we try not to categorize these foods as good or bad, when we eat mindfully we recognize that they may not be the best choices at all times. Mindful eating helps us to listen more closely to our inner voice and to make smart, sensible choices. Sometimes your inner voice will tell you that it's okay to eat a slice of cake—but more often than not, it will probably try to talk you into healthier fare. Listen to what it says and trust your instincts.

GREATER ENJOYMENT

The final principle of mindful eating is using your senses. When you get right down to it, eating food is fun! But since it is fun, we often overdo it, especially if we're distracted or feel unsatisfied with what we've already eaten. Food is also often associated with enjoyable experiences like birthday parties and backyard barbecues. Even something as simple as casually hanging out with friends often revolves around a food-based activity. Mindful eating teaches us to use all of our senses when we eat, and when you use all of your senses to enjoy a meal, it can help you to feel more satisfied with less food. Since eating is already an enjoyable activity, when you take the time to really pay attention to how food smells and tastes and feels, you end up feeling much more content with the experience.

While it's easier to engage all of your senses when you're not distracted, you can apply these principles when you're at a gathering or event to prevent yourself from inadvertently eating too much. Instead of simply eating your food without thought, pay attention to each bite. If you're having a conversation with someone, wait until you've completed a thought before taking another bite of your meal. You may find that you only need one plate of food at your next family get-together instead of going back for seconds.

> *"Always hold fast to the present. Every situation, indeed every moment, is of infinite value, for it is the representative of a whole eternity."*
>
> ~*Johann Wolfgang von Goethe, German poet and playwright*

INCORPORATING MINDFUL EATING INTO YOUR DAILY LIFE

START SLOWLY

We all lead busy lives and sometimes there's no way to prevent a rushed meal. So it's unrealistic to expect that we'll use the principles of mindful eating for every single meal we eat. At first, try to set aside one meal a week to practice mindful eating. Once you're used to the process, you can increase your mindful meals to a few times a week, or even once a day.

Many people find that lunchtime is the easiest time to practice mindful eating. In the morning, we're often rushing to get out the door to make it to work or school, and helping our families rush out the door as well. There isn't always time to slow down and enjoy breakfast. And in the evenings, we're tired, physically and mentally, and aren't always motivated to do much more than sit on the couch with some takeout and a favorite television program.

But lunch is often scheduled into our day, providing us with the perfect opportunity to take some time to slow down and practice mindful eating. Again, you don't need to eat every lunch in a mindful way, but try to choose one day when you can really unplug yourself from work or other responsibilities and pay attention to your meal.

SET A TIMER

Remember how it takes 20 minutes for your stomach to tell your brain that it's full? Use that as a guideline for your meal. Set a timer for 20 minutes, and use that entire time to mindfully eat your meal. This forces you to slow down and pay attention to each bite. And if you use the entire 20 minutes to eat your food, you'll give your body the time it needs to process the feeling of "fullness." Once you've hit the 20-minute mark, pause and think about how you feel. Are you full? Still hungry? Do you feel satisfied with the amount you've eaten or do you feel like you need more? Chances are, you'll feel content with the meal you've eaten and won't need to indulge any further.

EAT WITH YOUR NON-DOMINANT HAND

Have you ever tried to write your name or brush your teeth with your non-dominant hand? If you have, you know that it takes much longer to complete the task. Not only that, but you have to use much more concentration to will your hand to do what you want it to do. So when you sit down to practice mindful eating, use your non-dominant hand to hold your utensils and bring the food to your mouth. You'll be forced to eat much more slowly, and you'll automatically take smaller bites since it's easier to manipulate a smaller amount of food on a utensil when you're using a hand you're not used to using. Another trick you can try is to use chopsticks to eat your meal—this also requires more concentration and coordination, so you'll end up eating more slowly and can focus on every bite.

THINK ABOUT THE PROCESS

How often do you think about where your food comes from? Most of us can easily walk into a grocery store, pick up what we need, buy it and take it home, but those shelves at the grocery store are only part of the story. When you practice mindful eating, think about the people and the process that went into making your meal. We seldom think about just how much work goes into a meal from start to finish, but that food on your plate is the result of months of labor and care. Mindfully thinking about this process helps us to appreciate our meal even more and can also help us have gratitude for other things we're fortunate to have in our lives.

PAY ATTENTION TO HOW YOU FEEL

In many Asian cultures, there is a belief that one should eat until they are 80 percent full. Instead of continuing to eat until uncomfortably stuffed, diners pay attention to how they feel and make an effort to stop before reaching a point where their pants no longer button easily. By eating meals mindfully, we not only gauge our emotions and try to prevent eating because of how we mentally feel, but we also gauge our physical feelings. This can take some practice, since we're not always used to thinking about our physical state when we're enjoying a meal. But once you're tuned in to your physical feelings when you're eating, you will be better able to intuitively know when to stop eating in order to feel satisfied. You'll also feel better mentally, knowing that you've treated your body well.

TAKE SMALL BITES AND CHEW THOROUGHLY

Horace Fletcher may not have been right about all aspects of his diet advice—and chewing each bite 32 times is probably overkill—but he did have some ideas that can definitely be applied to mindful eating. When we eat without thought, not only do we eat too quickly, but we have a tendency to take bites that are too large and we chew those large bites too little. Not only does our meal disappear quickly, but the eating experience itself can be uncomfortable and unsatisfying. We don't even have time to register the tastes and textures of our food, or even appreciate the small break in our day that each meal provides. Instead of simply inhaling a meal as quickly as possible, we should deliberately take small bites and concentrate on chewing each bite thoroughly, taking the time you need to enjoy each bite.

PUT DOWN THE FORK

Instead of holding your utensils continuously throughout your meal, try putting your fork down between each bite. This is another trick that will force you to eat more slowly, simply because you'll be taking more time between bites to lift and lower your utensils. At first this may seem like a strange habit, but the point is to give you that small break between bites to think about the whole process. Whether you want to or not, you'll be slowing down when you eat in this manner, so it can be a great and simple routine to develop.

GETTING STARTED

Mindful eating can be a valuable tool to use to cultivate a healthier relationship with food. But with our busy lives, it's not always possible to sit down and quietly eat a meal in a mindful way. And families with kids may find it even more difficult— children aren't always likely to be interested in following rules and principles, especially if they're hungry and only interested in finding a snack. But it's important to remember that mindful eating doesn't need to be an all-or-nothing endeavor. Sometimes you won't be able to follow every single principle. You won't always be able to eat in total silence or find a place that is free of distractions. And sometimes you really do only have a few minutes to sneak in a meal.

But even when you're short on time or need to take care of your family's meals, you can incorporate concepts from the principles of mindful eating. Just take one or two ideas and use them to make quick meals or snacks more mindful, even when you don't have the time or concentration for a more thoughtful session.

For instance, to make mindful eating a bit more fun for kids, try a new fruit together. Grocery stores often have specialty varieties like dragon fruit, star fruit or lychee fruit. Have your child pick out something new to try, and then examine and sample it together. You may find that your kids look forward to grocery trips to pick out new foods to try!

Another simple and easy mindful eating strategy you can try with your family is to ask everyone to eat in silence for the first few minutes of a meal. Tell them to think about where the food came from and about all the people who worked to make the meal. Talk about how fortunate we are to have access to the food we eat, and how grateful we should be for all the people who work hard to provide us with nourishing meals. In this way, your whole family can be more mindful when they eat together.

If you're eating with a friend, you can add a bit of mindfulness as well. Instead of focusing all your attention on talking without paying attention to your food, make sure to stop talking when you take a bite of your meal. Sharing a meal offers us an opportunity to practice mindfulness by listening to our friends, while also being aware of the food we eat. You could even ask your friend to join you in a mindful meal, by taking bites in silence and talking between bites.

And if you're eating alone, there are other simple ideas you can use. When we're alone, many of us don't like to simply sit and eat in silence—often we watch television or read a book. But you can still have some moments of mindful eating. If you watch a television show while eating, hit the pause button or put the television on mute while you take a couple bites of your meal. If you're reading a book, read a page and then close the book and take a bite of food. Then alternate back to reading a page. In this way, even when you have distractions nearby, you can still focus all of your attention on each bite of food.

With our busy lives, we don't often have the time or the energy to really plan out healthy meals and snacks. We grab food and go, not even thinking about what we're eating. And often times it's gone before we even realize we've eaten anything. Mindful eating helps us to make better choices, to think about what kinds foods we put in our bodies, and to consider how much food we eat. We can eat less food but be more satisfied, while enjoying all the tastes, smells, and textures we experience. The best thing about incorporating mindful eating into your routine is that you'll live a healthier, more fulfilling lifestyle—and all you have to do is eat!

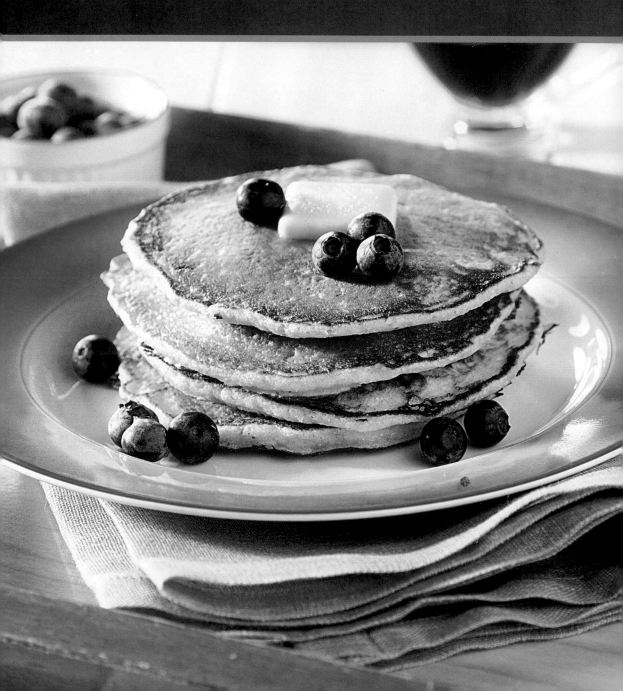

BREAKFAST

CORNMEAL PANCAKES

2 cups buttermilk

2 eggs, lightly beaten

¼ cup sugar

2 tablespoons butter, melted

1½ cups yellow cornmeal

¾ cup all-purpose flour

1½ teaspoons baking powder

1 teaspoon salt

Fresh blueberries, butter and maple syrup (optional)

1. Beat buttermilk, eggs, sugar and butter in large bowl until well blended. Combine cornmeal, flour, baking powder and salt in medium bowl; mix well. Stir into buttermilk mixture until blended. Let stand 5 minutes.

2. Lightly grease griddle or large skillet; heat over medium heat. Pour batter onto griddle ⅓ cup at a time. Cook 3 minutes or until tops of pancakes are bubbly and appear dry; turn and cook 2 minutes or until bottoms are golden brown. Serve with blueberries, butter and maple syrup, if desired.

MAKES 4 SERVINGS

MEDITERRANEAN
ARTICHOKE OMELET

2 eggs

1 tablespoon grated Parmesan
   cheese

2 tablespoons olive oil

3 drained canned artichoke
   bottoms, diced

1 ounce (about 2 pieces)
   roasted red bell pepper,
   diced

½ teaspoon minced garlic

1 tablespoon tomato salsa

1. Beat eggs in small bowl. Stir in cheese.

2. Heat oil in large nonstick skillet over medium-high heat. Add artichokes; cook and stir 2 to 3 minutes or until beginning to brown. Add roasted pepper; cook and stir 2 minutes or until liquid has evaporated. Add garlic; cook and stir 30 seconds. Remove to small plate; keep warm.

3. Add egg mixture to skillet. Lift edge of omelet with spatula to allow uncooked portion to flow underneath. Cook 1 to 2 minutes or until omelet is almost set.

4. Spoon artichoke mixture onto half of omelet; fold omelet over filling. Cook 2 minutes until set. Serve with salsa.

MAKES 1 SERVING

Note: Raw eggs will turn green if combined with raw artichokes because of a chemical reaction between the two foods. Cooking the artichokes separately will prevent this from happening.

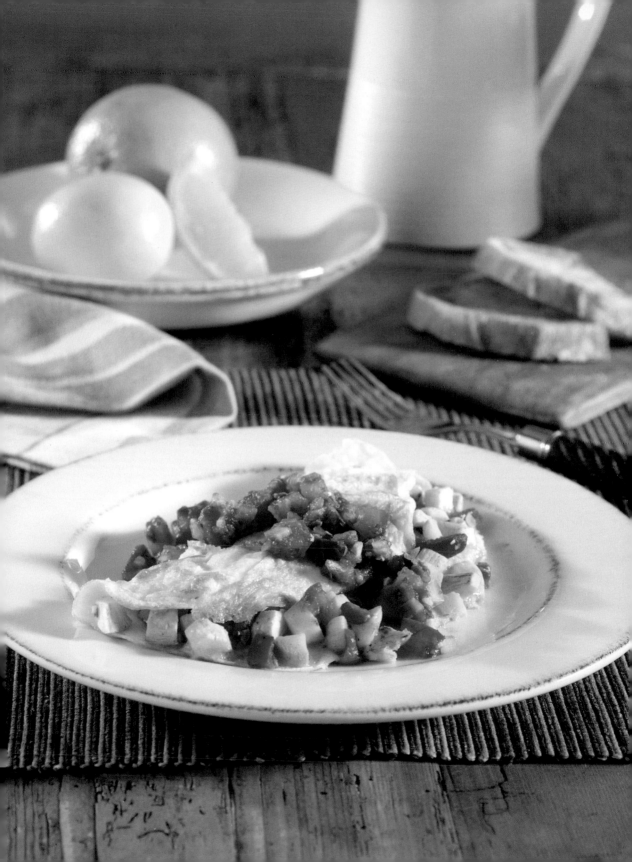

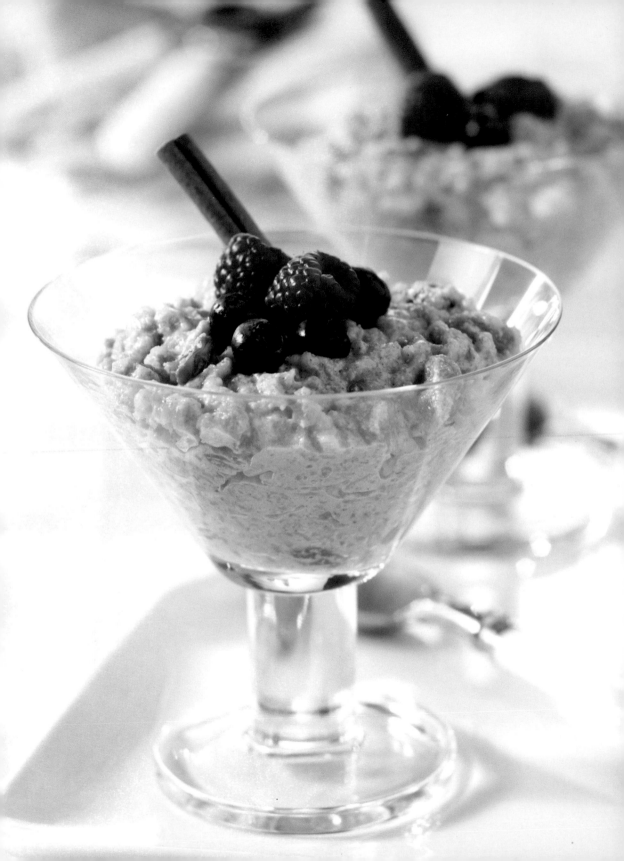

BREAKFAST RICE PUDDING

2 cups vanilla soymilk, divided

¾ cup quick-cooking brown rice*

⅓ cup packed brown sugar

½ teaspoon ground cinnamon

½ teaspoon salt

¼ cup golden raisins or dried sweetened cranberries (optional)

½ teaspoon vanilla

Mixed berries (optional)

*Look for rice that cooks in 20 to 25 minutes. For rice with a longer cooking time, increase the cooking time in step 1.

1. Bring 1½ cups soymilk to a simmer in medium saucepan over medium heat. Stir in rice, brown sugar, cinnamon and salt; cover and simmer 10 minutes.

2. Stir in remaining ½ cup soymilk and raisins, if desired; cover and simmer 10 minutes. Remove from heat; stir in vanilla. Serve with berries, if desired.

MAKES 4 SERVINGS

Note: Rice thickens as it cools. For a thinner consistency, stir in additional soymilk just before serving.

BLUEBERRY BANANA OATMEAL SMOOTHIE »

1 cup milk

1 banana

½ cup frozen blueberries

½ cup plain Greek yogurt

¼ cup quick oats

1. Combine milk, banana and blueberries in blender; blend until smooth. Add yogurt and oats; blend until smooth.

2. Pour into 2 glasses. Serve immediately.

MAKES 2 SERVINGS

MANGO-GINGER SMOOTHIE

2½ cups sliced peeled fresh peaches *or* 1 package (16 ounces) frozen sliced peaches

2½ cups cubed fresh or jarred mango

1 container (6 ounces) vanilla yogurt

2 tablespoons honey

2 teaspoons fresh grated ginger

1 cup ice cubes

1. Combine peaches, mango, yogurt, honey, ginger and ice in blender; blend until smooth.

2. Pour into 4 glasses. Serve immediately.

MAKES 4 SERVINGS

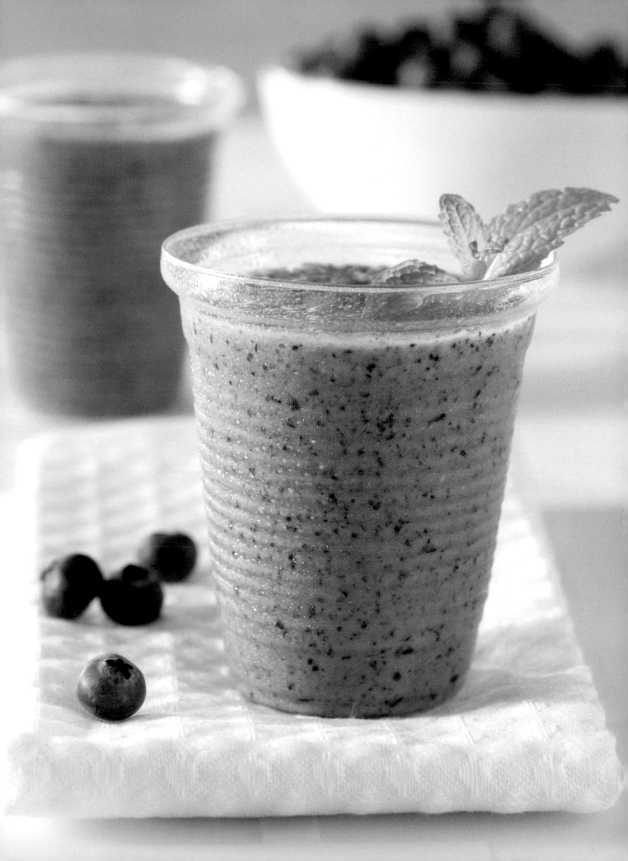

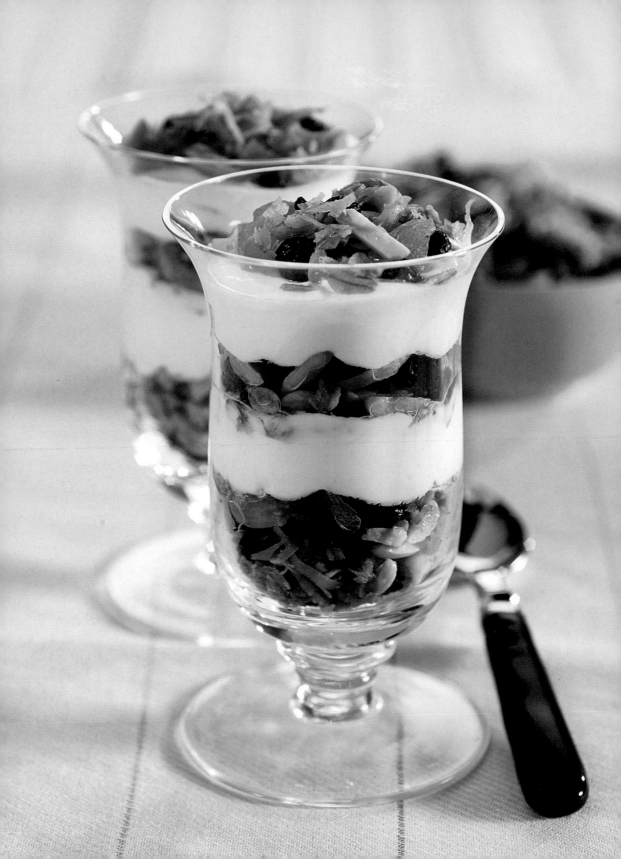

CHUNKY FRUITY HOMEMADE GRANOLA

2 cups old-fashioned oats

1⅓ cups raw slivered almonds

1 cup shredded coconut

3 tablespoons butter

¼ cup honey

1 cup dried apricots, chopped

¾ cup dried cranberries

¾ cup dried tart cherries

½ cup dried blueberries

½ cup roasted unsalted cashew pieces

1. Preheat oven to 300°F. Line baking sheet with foil or parchment paper.

2. Combine oats, almonds and coconut in large bowl. Place butter in small microwavable bowl; microwave on HIGH 30 to 45 seconds or until melted. Whisk in honey until blended. Pour butter mixture over oat mixture; toss to coat. Spread on prepared baking sheet.

3. Bake 20 to 25 minutes or until golden, stirring once or twice during baking. Cool mixture on baking sheet on wire rack.

4. Combine apricots, cranberries, cherries, blueberries and cashews in large bowl. Crumble cooled oat mixture into fruit mixture; stir until blended.

MAKES ABOUT 8 CUPS

Serving Suggestions: Layer the granola with a cup of yogurt for a quick breakfast parfait. It can be served as a snack on its own, or as part of a dessert sprinkled over ice cream or frozen yogurt. Keep it stored in an airtight container to maintain its crispiness.

FETA BRUNCH BAKE

1 medium red bell pepper

2 packages (10 ounces each) fresh spinach, stemmed

6 eggs

1½ cups (6 ounces) crumbled feta cheese

⅓ cup chopped onion

2 tablespoons chopped fresh parsley

¼ teaspoon dried dill weed

Dash black pepper

1. Preheat broiler. Place bell pepper on foil-lined broiler pan. Broil 4 inches from heat source 15 to 20 minutes or until blackened on all sides, turning every 5 minutes with tongs. Place in paper bag; close bag and set aside to cool 15 to 20 minutes. Cut out core and remove seeds. Cut roasted pepper in half and rub off skin; rinse under cold water. Cut into ½-inch pieces.

2. Fill medium saucepan half full with water; bring to a boil over high heat. Add spinach and return to a boil; boil 2 to 3 minutes or until wilted. Drain and immediately plunge into bowl of cold water to stop cooking. Drain spinach; let stand until cool enough to handle. Squeeze to remove excess water; finely chop.

3. Preheat oven to 400°F. Spray 1-quart baking dish with nonstick cooking spray.

4. Beat eggs in large bowl until foamy. Stir in roasted pepper, spinach, cheese, onion, parsley, dill and black pepper. Pour into prepared baking dish.

5. Bake 20 minutes or until set. Let stand 5 minutes before serving.

MAKES 4 SERVINGS

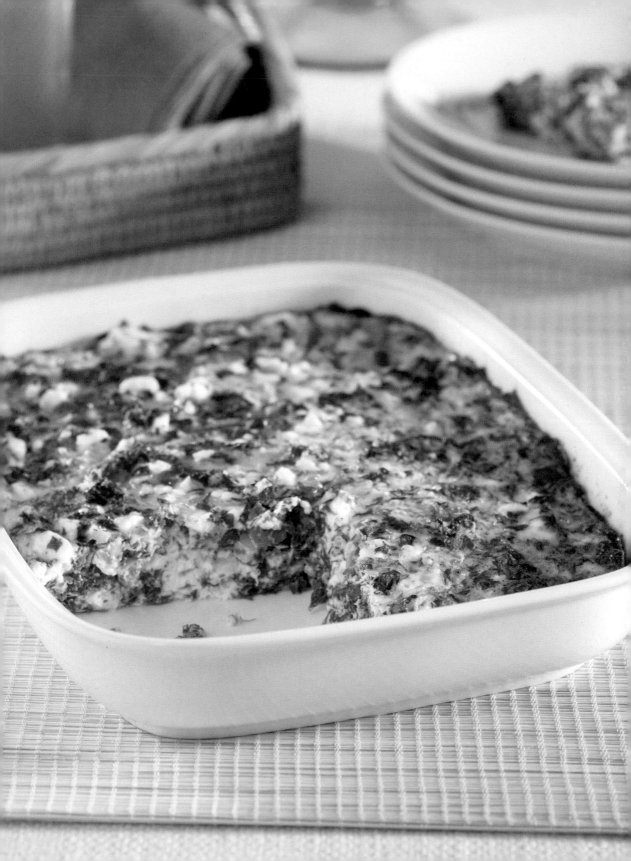

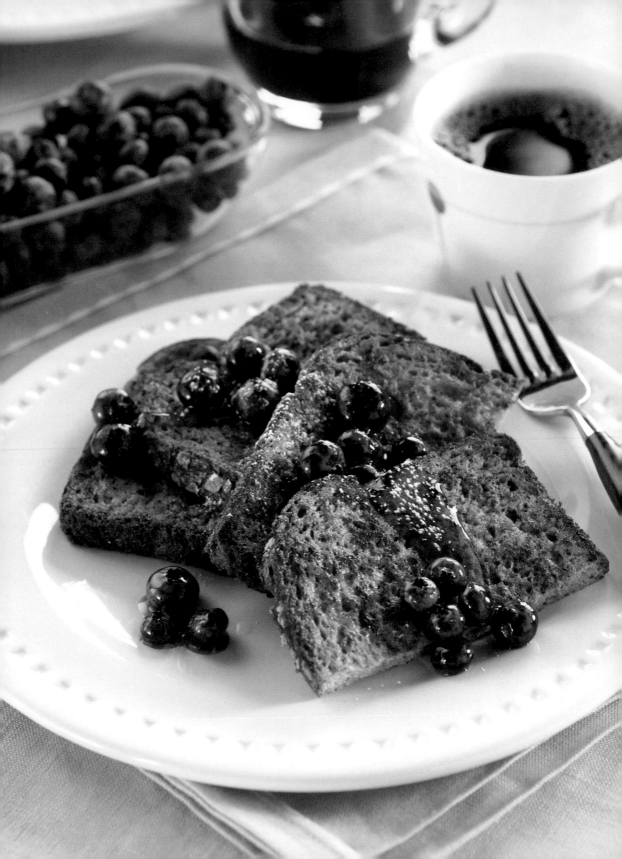

WHOLE GRAIN FRENCH TOAST

2 eggs

¼ cup milk

½ teaspoon ground cinnamon

¼ teaspoon ground nutmeg

4 teaspoons butter

8 slices whole wheat or multigrain bread

⅓ cup pure maple syrup

1 cup fresh blueberries

Powdered sugar (optional)

1. Preheat oven to 400°F. Spray baking sheet with nonstick cooking spray.

2. Beat eggs, milk, cinnamon and nutmeg in shallow bowl until well blended. Melt 1 teaspoon butter in large nonstick skillet over medium heat. Dip 2 bread slices in egg mixture, turning to coat; let excess drip back into bowl. Cook 2 minutes per side or until golden brown. Transfer to prepared baking sheet. Repeat with remaining butter, bread slices and egg mixture.

3. Bake 5 to 6 minutes or until heated through.

4. Place maple syrup in small microwavable bowl; microwave on HIGH 30 seconds or until bubbly. Stir in blueberries. Serve French toast with syrup mixture; sprinkle with powdered sugar, if desired.

MAKES 4 SERVINGS

SIMPLE BREAKFAST SANDWICHES

3 eggs

¼ teaspoon salt

¼ teaspoon black pepper *or*
   ⅛ teaspoon hot pepper sauce

3 slices (2 ounces) Canadian
   bacon, chopped

1 green onion, thinly sliced

2 teaspoons butter

⅓ cup shredded sharp
   Cheddar cheese

4 multigrain or whole wheat
   English muffins, split
   and toasted

1. Beat eggs, salt and pepper in medium bowl until blended. Stir in Canadian bacon and green onion.

2. Heat butter in medium nonstick skillet over medium-high heat until bubbly. Add egg mixture; cook 2 to 3 minutes or until eggs are soft-set, stirring frequently. Remove from heat; stir in cheese. Serve on English muffins.

MAKES 4 SERVINGS

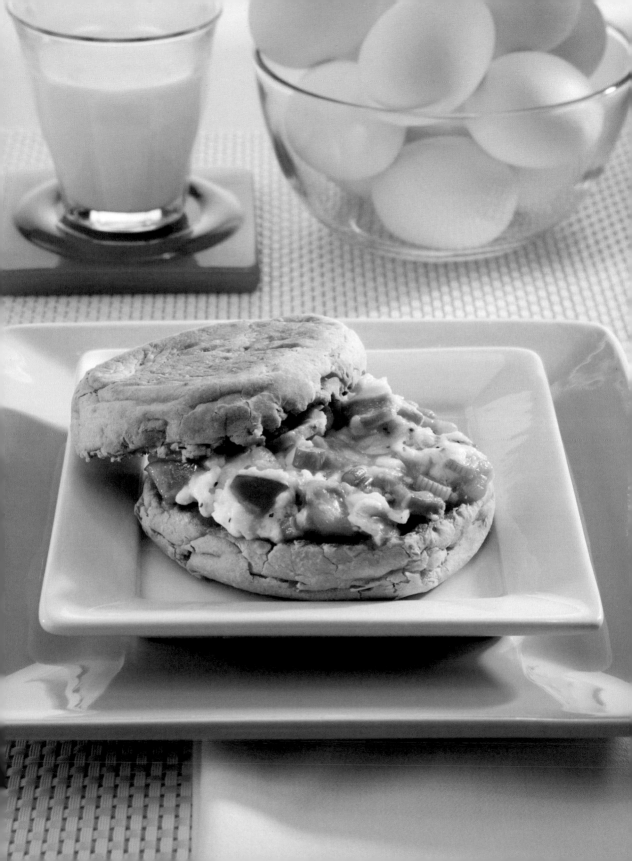

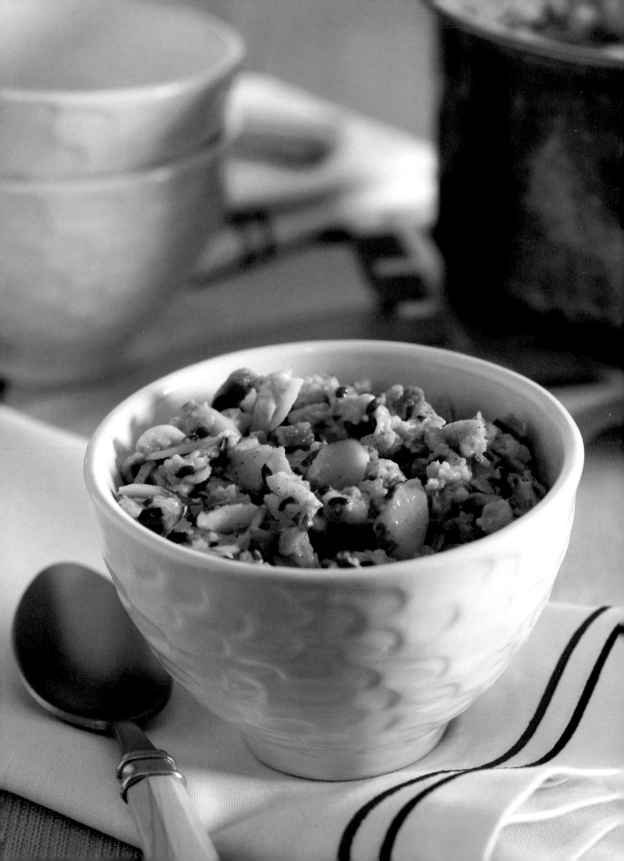

SUPER OATMEAL

2 cups water

2¾ cups old-fashioned oats

½ cup finely diced dried figs*

⅓ cup lightly packed dark
brown sugar

⅓ to ½ cup sliced almonds,
toasted**

¼ cup flaxseeds

½ teaspoon salt

½ teaspoon ground cinnamon

2 cups milk, plus additional
for serving

*Beige Turkish figs are recommended
if your market carries them.

**To toast almonds, cook in medium
skillet over medium heat 1 to 2 minutes
or until lightly browned, stirring frequently.

1. Bring water to a boil in large saucepan over high heat. Stir in oats, figs, brown sugar, almonds, flaxseeds, salt and cinnamon. Immediately add 2 cups milk; mix well.

2. Reduce heat to medium-high; cook and stir 5 to 7 minutes or until oatmeal is thick and creamy. Serve with additional milk, if desired.

MAKES 5 TO 6 SERVINGS

TROPICAL FRUIT BREAKFAST PARFAITS

4 containers (6 ounces each) vanilla yogurt

1 banana, mashed

2 tablespoons maple syrup

¾ to 1 teaspoon ground cinnamon

1 cup oat flakes cereal

½ cup flaked coconut

1 can (8 ounces) crushed pineapple in juice, drained

2 cups fresh strawberries, quartered

1 kiwi, peeled and diced

1. Combine yogurt, banana, maple syrup and cinnamon in medium bowl; mix well.

2. Spoon about ⅓ cup yogurt mixture into each of 4 parfait or wine glasses; top with cereal, coconut and fruit.

MAKES 4 SERVINGS

Variations: Substitute plain yogurt for vanilla yogurt. Substitute honey for maple syrup.

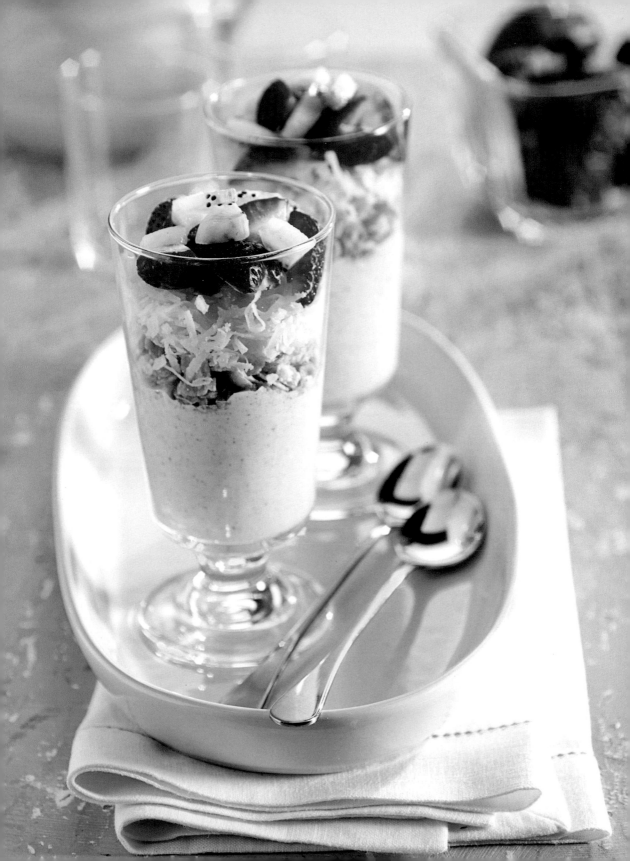

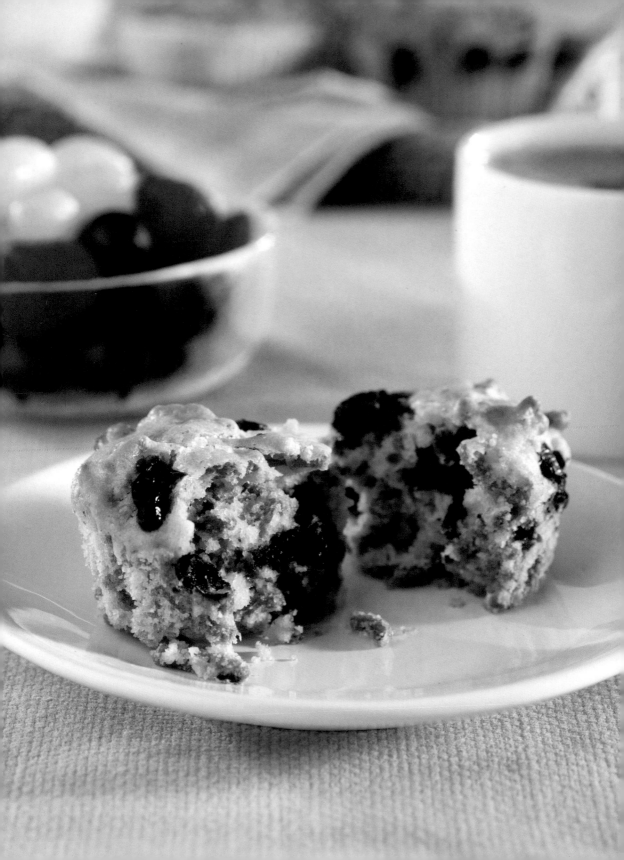

BERRY BRAN MUFFINS

2 cups dry bran cereal

1¼ cups milk

½ cup packed brown sugar

¼ cup coconut oil

1 egg, lightly beaten

1 teaspoon vanilla

1¼ cups all-purpose flour

1 tablespoon baking powder

¼ teaspoon salt

1 cup fresh or frozen blueberries (partially thawed if frozen)

1. Preheat oven to 350°F. Line 12 standard (2¾-inch) muffin cups with paper baking cups.

2. Combine cereal and milk in medium bowl; mix well. Let stand 5 minutes to soften. Add brown sugar, oil, egg and vanilla; beat until well blended.

3. Combine flour, baking powder and salt in large bowl; mix well. Add cereal mixture; stir just until dry ingredients are moistened. Gently fold in blueberries. Spoon batter into prepared muffin cups, filling almost full.

4. Bake 20 to 25 minutes (25 to 30 if using frozen berries) or until toothpick inserted into centers comes out clean. Serve warm.

MAKES 12 SERVINGS

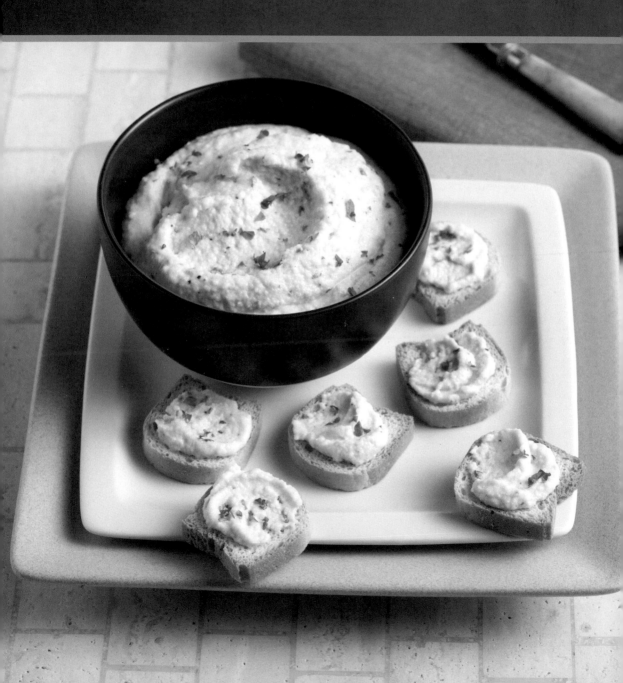

SNACKS

CREAMY CASHEW SPREAD

1 cup raw cashew nuts

2 tablespoons lemon juice

1 tablespoon tahini

½ teaspoon salt

½ teaspoon black pepper

2 teaspoons minced fresh herbs, such as basil, parsley or oregano (optional)

Assorted bread toasts and/or crackers

1. Rinse cashews; place in medium bowl. Cover with water by at least 2 inches; soak 4 hours or overnight. Drain cashews, reserving soaking water.

2. Place cashews, 2 tablespoons reserved water, lemon juice, tahini, salt and pepper in food processor or blender; process several minutes or until smooth. Add additional water, 1 tablespoon at a time, until desired consistency is reached.

3. Cover and refrigerate until ready to serve. Stir in herbs, if desired, just before serving. Serve with assorted bread toasts and/or crackers.

MAKES ABOUT ½ CUP (6 SERVINGS)

Serving Suggestions: Use as a spread or dip for hors d'oeuvres, or as a sandwich spread or pasta topping. Thin with additional liquid as needed.

FRUITED GRANOLA

3 cups quick oats

1 cup sliced almonds

1 cup honey

½ cup wheat germ

3 tablespoons butter, melted

1 teaspoon ground cinnamon

3 cups whole grain cereal flakes

½ cup dried blueberries
or golden raisins

½ cup dried cranberries
or cherries

½ cup dried banana chips
or chopped pitted dates

1. Preheat oven to 325°F.

2. Spread oats and almonds in 13×9-inch baking pan. Bake 15 minutes or until lightly toasted, stirring frequently.

3. Combine honey, wheat germ, butter and cinnamon in large bowl; mix well. Add oats and almonds; toss to coat. Spread mixture in same baking pan; bake 20 minutes or until golden brown. Remove to wire rack to cool completely. Break mixture into chunks.

4. Combine oat chunks, cereal, blueberries, cranberries and banana chips in large bowl. Store in airtight container at room temperature up to 2 weeks.

MAKES ABOUT 10 CUPS

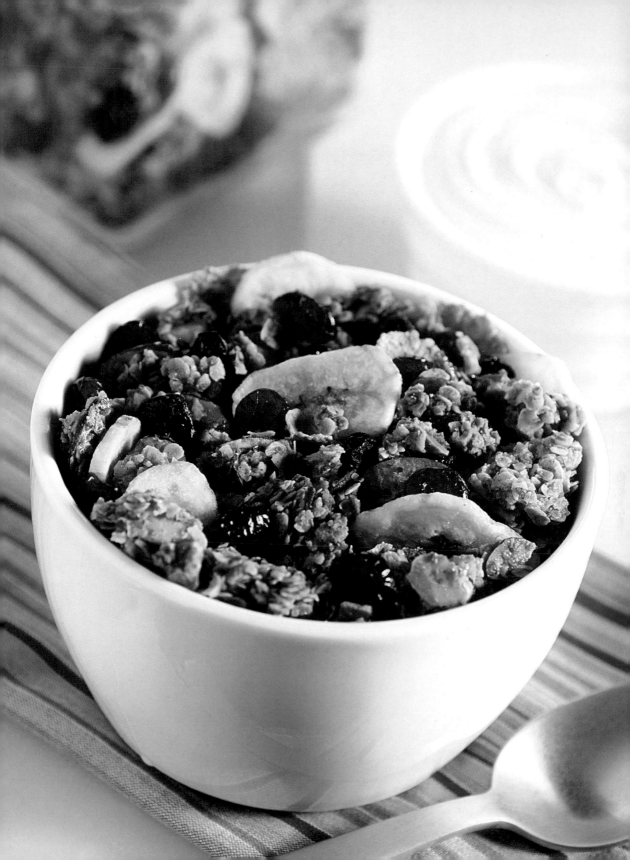

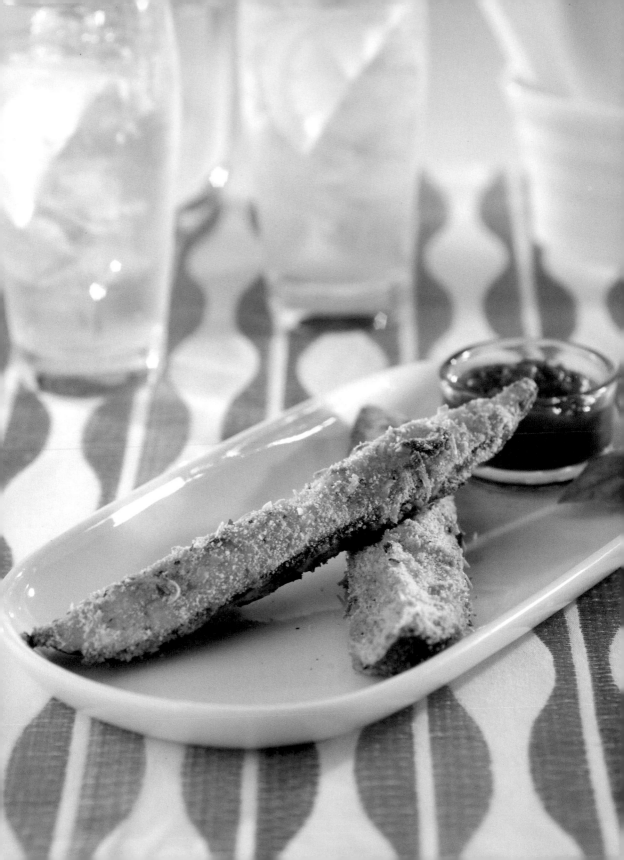

SAVORY ZUCCHINI STIX

3 tablespoons seasoned dry
   bread crumbs

2 tablespoons grated Parmesan
   cheese

1 egg

1 teaspoon milk

2 small zucchini (about
   4 ounces each), cut
   lengthwise into quarters

⅓ cup pasta sauce, warmed

1. Preheat oven to 400°F. Spray baking sheet with nonstick cooking spray.

2. Combine bread crumbs and cheese in shallow dish; mix well. Beat egg and milk in another shallow dish until well blended.

3. Dip each zucchini wedge first in crumb mixture, then in egg white mixture, letting excess drip back into dish. Roll again in crumb mixture to coat. Place zucchini sticks on prepared baking sheet.

4. Bake 15 to 18 minutes or until golden brown. Serve with pasta sauce for dipping.

MAKES 4 SERVINGS

LITTLE LEMON BASIL POPS

1¼ cups plain Greek yogurt

¼ cup milk

Grated peel and juice of
  1 lemon

2 tablespoons sugar

2 tablespoons chopped
  fresh basil

Ice cube trays

Pop sticks

1. Combine yogurt, milk, lemon peel, lemon juice, sugar and basil in blender or food processor; blend until smooth.

2. Pour mixture into ice cube trays. Freeze 2 hours.

3. Insert sticks. Freeze 4 to 6 hours or until firm.

4. To remove pops from trays, place bottoms of ice cube trays under warm running water until loosened. Press firmly on bottoms to release. (Do not twist or pull sticks.)

MAKES 16 POPS

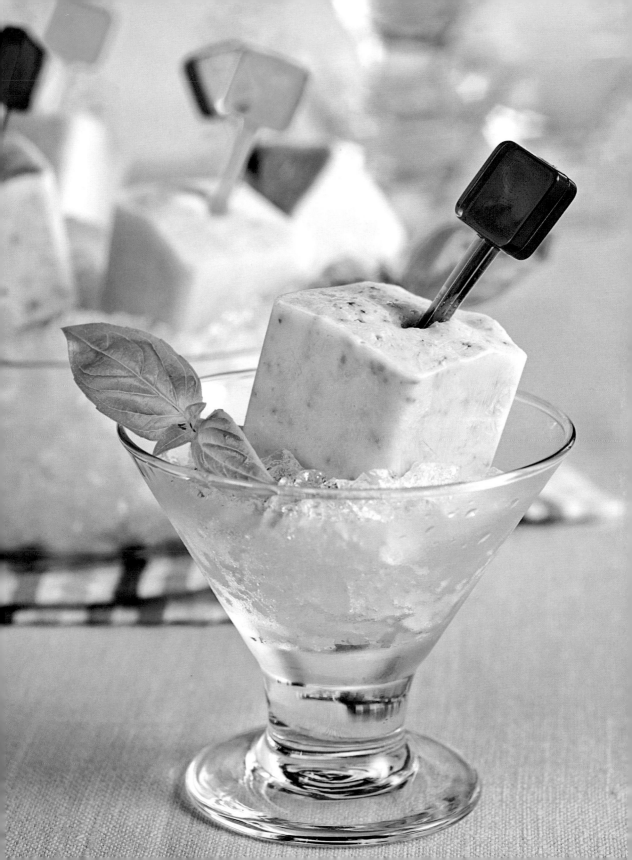

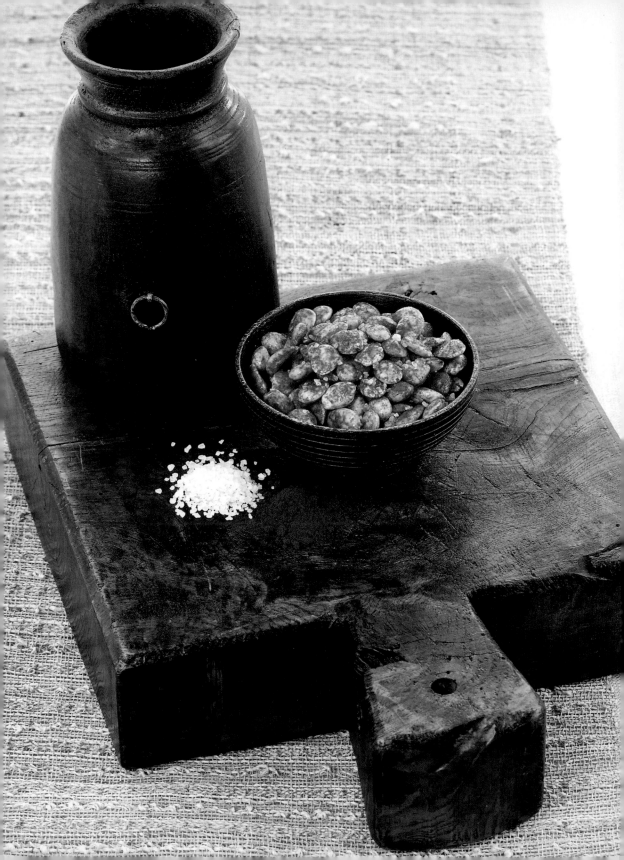

« PAPRIKA-SPICED ALMONDS

1 cup whole blanched almonds
1 teaspoon extra virgin olive oil
¼ teaspoon coarse salt

¼ teaspoon smoked paprika
   or paprika

1. Preheat oven to 375°F. Spread almonds in single layer in shallow baking pan.

2. Bake 8 to 10 minutes or until almonds are lightly browned. Transfer to bowl; cool 5 minutes. Drizzle with oil; toss to coat. Sprinkle with salt and paprika; toss again.

MAKES ABOUT 4 SERVINGS

Tip: For the best flavor, serve these almonds the day they are made.

BITE-YOU-BACK ROASTED EDAMAME

2 teaspoons vegetable oil
2 teaspoons honey
¼ teaspoon wasabi powder*
1 package (10 ounces) shelled edamame, thawed if frozen

Coarse salt (optional)

*Wasabi powder can be found in the Asian section of most supermarkets and in Asian specialty markets.

1. Preheat oven to 375°F.

2. Combine oil, honey and wasabi powder in large bowl; mix well. Add edamame; toss to coat. Spread in single layer on baking sheet.

3. Bake 12 to 15 minutes or until golden brown, stirring once. Immediately remove from baking sheet to large bowl; sprinkle generously with salt, if desired. Cool completely before serving. Store in airtight container.

MAKES 4 TO 6 SERVINGS

GUACAMOLE

2 large avocados

¼ cup finely chopped tomato, plus additional for garnish

2 tablespoons fresh lime juice or lemon juice

2 tablespoons grated onion with juice

½ teaspoon salt

¼ teaspoon hot pepper sauce

Black pepper

1. Place avocados in medium bowl; mash coarsely with fork. Stir in ¼ cup tomato, lime juice, onion with juice, salt, hot pepper sauce and black pepper; mix well.

2. Serve immediately or cover and refrigerate up to 2 hours. Garnish with additional tomato.

MAKES 2 CUPS

Tip: To ripen firm avocados, store them in a loosely closed paper bag at room temperature for a few days.

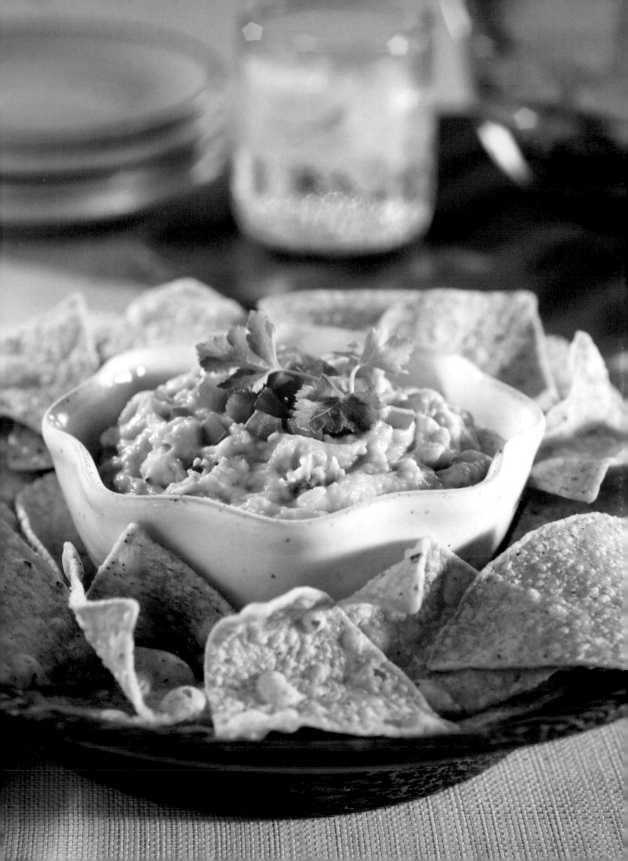

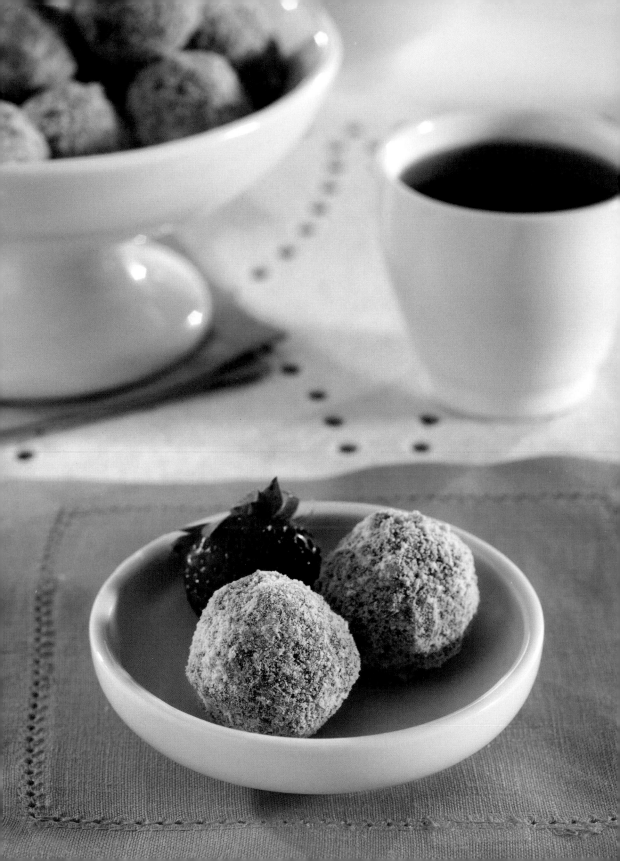

TRAIL MIX TRUFFLES

⅓ cup dried apples

¼ cup dried apricots

¼ cup apple butter

2 tablespoons golden raisins

1 tablespoon peanut butter

½ cup granola

¼ cup graham cracker crumbs, divided

¼ cup mini chocolate chips

1 tablespoon water

1. Combine apples, apricots, apple butter, raisins and peanut butter in food processor or blender; process until smooth.

2. Stir in granola, 1 tablespoon graham cracker crumbs, chocolate chips and water until well blended. Shape mixture into 16 balls.

3. Place remaining graham cracker crumbs in shallow dish; roll balls in crumbs to coat. Cover and refrigerate until ready to serve.

MAKES 8 SERVINGS

PURPLE PICK-ME-UP »

¼ cup water

1 navel orange, peeled
   and seeded

1 cup frozen blueberries

4 Medjool dates, pitted

1. Combine water, orange, blueberries and dates in blender; blend until smooth.

2. Pour into 2 glasses. Serve immediately.

MAKES 2 SERVINGS

ENERGY SMOOTHIE

1 package (16 ounces) frozen
   strawberries, partially thawed

2 medium ripe bananas

1 container (6 ounces) lemon
   or vanilla yogurt

1 cup milk

2 tablespoons honey

2 teaspoons vanilla

1. Combine strawberries, bananas, yogurt, milk, honey and vanilla in blender; blend until smooth.

2. Pour into 4 glasses. Serve immediately.

MAKES 4 SERVINGS

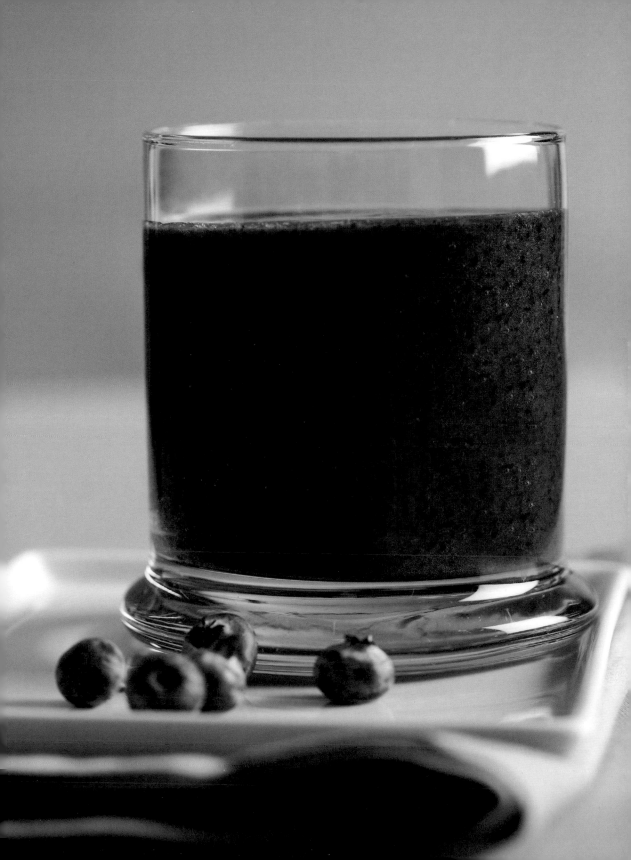

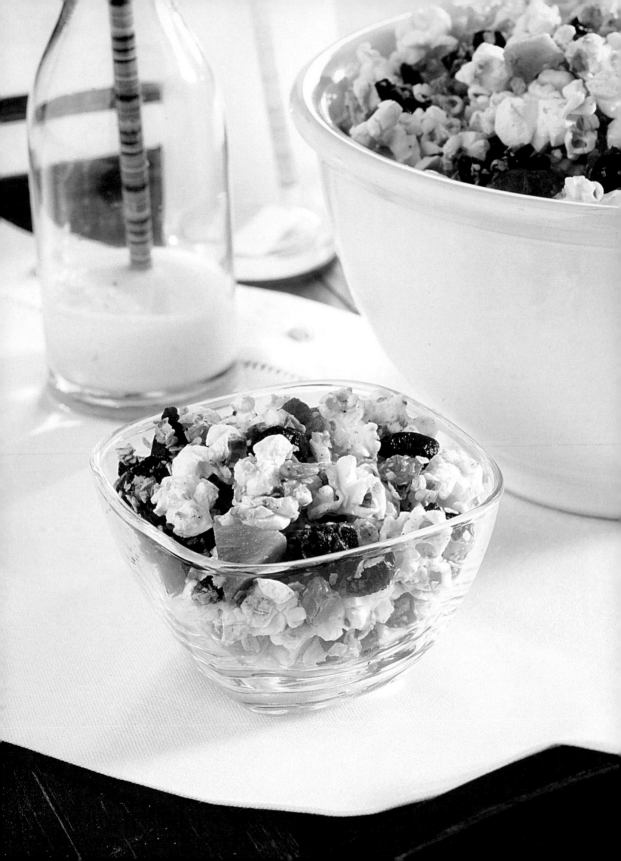

POPCORN GRANOLA

1 cup quick oats

6 cups air-popped popcorn

1 cup golden raisins

½ cup chopped mixed dried fruit

¼ cup sunflower kernels

2 tablespoons butter

2 tablespoons packed brown sugar

1 tablespoon honey

¼ teaspoon ground cinnamon

¼ teaspoon ground nutmeg

1. Preheat oven to 350°F. Spread oats on ungreased baking sheet; bake 10 to 15 minutes or until lightly toasted, stirring occasionally.

2. Combine oats, popcorn, raisins, dried fruit and sunflower kernels in large bowl; mix well.

3. Combine butter, brown sugar, honey, cinnamon and nutmeg in small saucepan; cook and stir over medium heat until butter is melted. Drizzle over popcorn mixture; toss to coat.

MAKES 8 SERVINGS

QUICK AND EASY HUMMUS

1 clove garlic, peeled

1 can (about 15 ounces) chickpeas, rinsed and drained

2 tablespoons torn fresh mint leaves (optional)

2 tablespoons olive oil

2 tablespoons lemon juice

2 teaspoons dark sesame oil

½ teaspoon salt

⅛ teaspoon ground red pepper or ¼ teaspoon hot pepper sauce

1. With motor running, drop garlic clove through feed tube of food processor; process until garlic is finely chopped.

2. Add chickpeas, mint, if desired, olive oil, lemon juice, sesame oil, salt and red pepper; process until hummus is smooth.

MAKES 4 SERVINGS

Serving Suggestion: Serve with vegetable dippers or pita wedges.

Tip: Leftover hummus may be covered and refrigerated up to 1 week. Hummus makes a great sandwich spread for pitas.

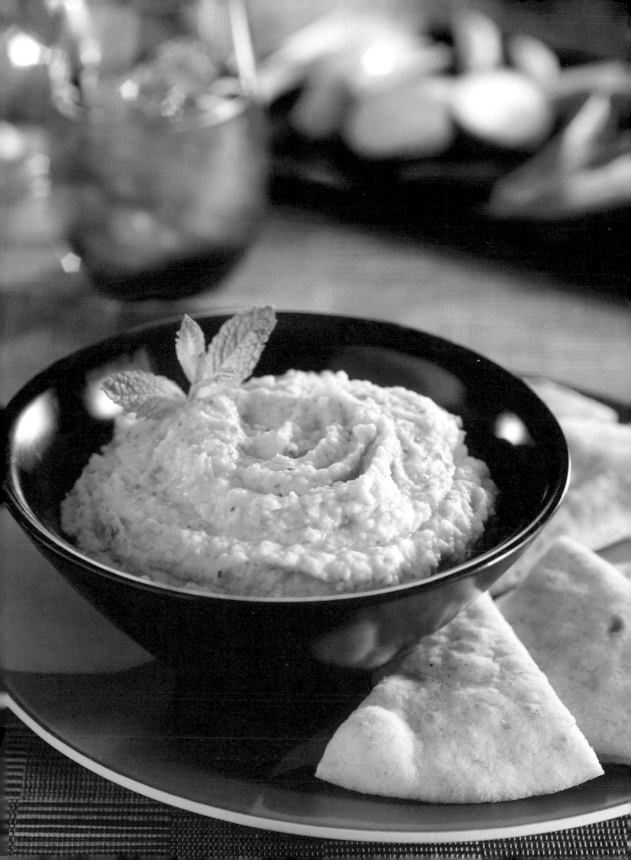

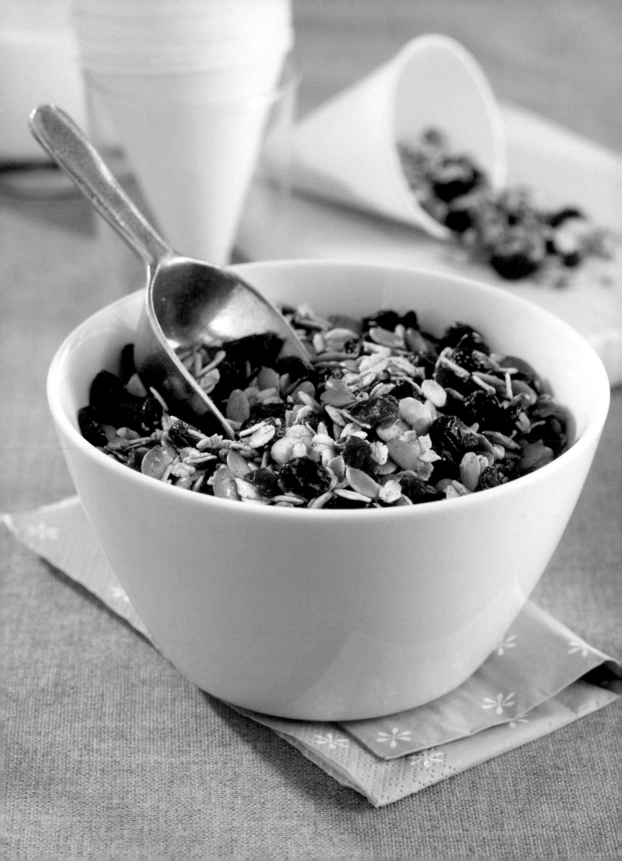

CRISP OATS TRAIL MIX

1 cup old-fashioned oats

½ cup unsalted shelled pumpkin
    seeds

½ cup dried cranberries

½ cup raisins

2 tablespoons maple syrup

1 tablespoon coconut oil

½ teaspoon ground cinnamon

¼ teaspoon salt

1. Preheat oven to 325°F. Line baking sheet with heavy-duty foil.

2. Combine oats, pumpkin seeds, cranberries, raisins, maple syrup, oil, cinnamon and salt in large bowl; mix well. Spread on prepared baking sheet.

3. Bake 20 minutes or until oats are lightly browned, stirring halfway through cooking time. Cool completely on baking sheet. Store in airtight container.

MAKES 2½ CUPS (ABOUT 10 SERVINGS)

SAVORY PITA CHIPS

2 whole wheat or white pita
  bread rounds

1 tablespoon olive oil

3 tablespoons grated Parmesan
  cheese

1 teaspoon dried basil

¼ teaspoon garlic powder

1. Preheat oven to 350°F. Line baking sheet with foil.

2. Carefully cut each pita round in half horizontally; split into 2 rounds.
Cut each round into 6 wedges.

3. Place pita wedges on prepared baking sheet; brush lightly with oil
on both sides.

4. Combine cheese, basil and garlic powder in small bowl; mix well.
Sprinkle evenly over pita wedges.

5. Bake 12 to 14 minutes or until golden brown. Cool completely.

MAKES 4 SERVINGS

Cinnamon Crisps: Substitute butter for the olive oil and 1 tablespoon sugar
mixed with ¼ teaspoon ground cinnamon for Parmesan cheese, basil and garlic
powder.

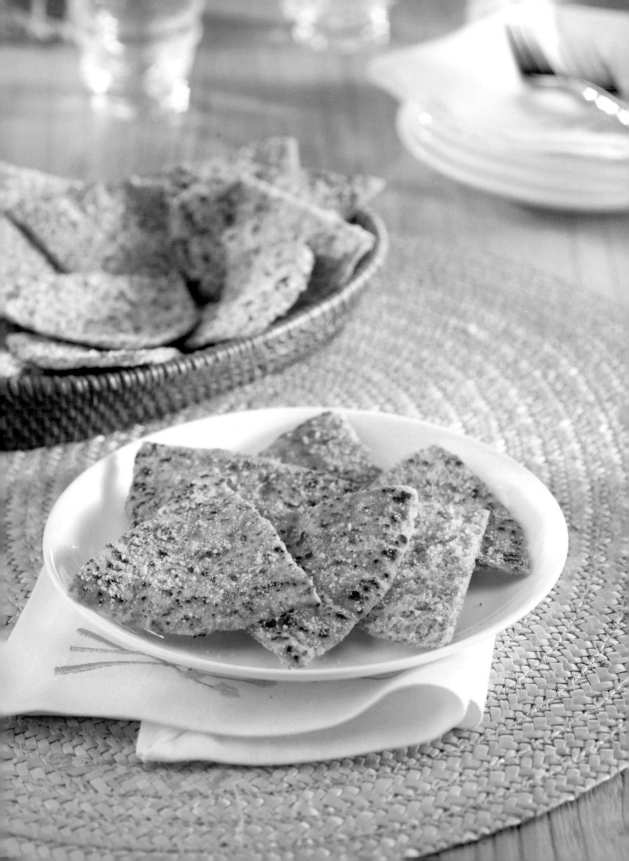

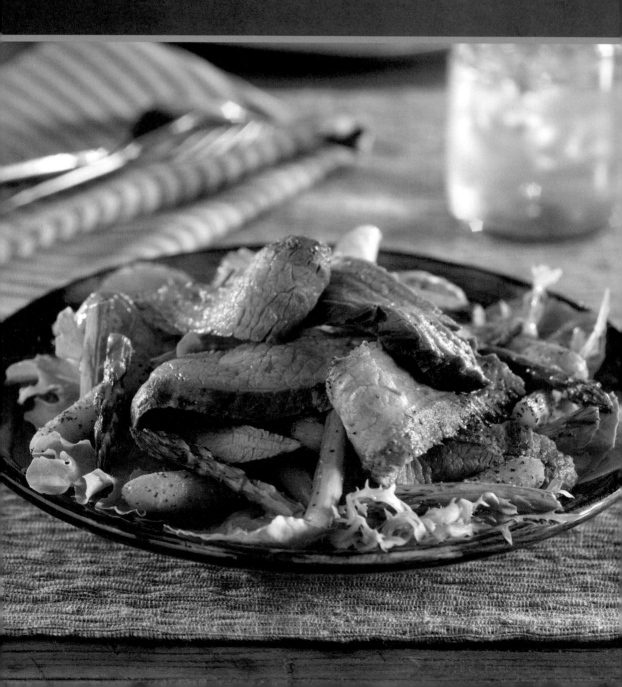

SALADS

FLANK STEAK AND ROASTED VEGETABLE SALAD

1½ pounds asparagus spears, trimmed and cut into 2-inch lengths

1¾ cups baby carrots (8 ounces)

2 tablespoons olive oil, divided

¾ teaspoon salt, divided

1 teaspoon black pepper, divided

1 pound flank steak (1 inch thick)

2 tablespoons plus 1 teaspoon Dijon mustard, divided

1 tablespoon fresh lemon juice

1 tablespoon water

1 teaspoon honey

6 cups mixed salad greens

1. Preheat oven to 400°F. Place asparagus and carrots in shallow roasting pan. Add 1 tablespoon oil, ¼ teaspoon salt and ¼ teaspoon pepper; toss to coat.

2. Roast 20 minutes or until vegetables are browned and tender, stirring once. Meanwhile, sprinkle steak with ¼ teaspoon salt and ½ teaspoon pepper. Rub both sides of steak with 2 tablespoons mustard. Place steak on rack in baking pan.

3. Roast steak 10 minutes for medium rare or to desired doneness, turning once. Let stand 5 minutes before cutting across the grain into thin slices.

4. Whisk lemon juice, remaining 1 tablespoon oil, water, honey, remaining 1 teaspoon mustard, ¼ teaspoon salt and ¼ teaspoon pepper in large bowl until well blended. Drizzle 1 tablespoon dressing over vegetables in pan; toss to coat. Add greens to dressing remaining in bowl; toss to coat. Divide greens among serving plates; top with steak and vegetables.

MAKES 4 SERVINGS

LENTIL AND ORZO PASTA SALAD

8 cups water

½ cup dried lentils, rinsed and sorted

4 ounces uncooked orzo

1½ cups quartered cherry or grape tomatoes

¾ cup finely chopped celery

½ cup chopped red onion

2 ounces pitted olives (about 16 olives), coarsely chopped

3 to 4 tablespoons cider vinegar

1 tablespoon olive oil

1 tablespoon dried basil

1 clove garlic, minced

⅛ teaspoon red pepper flakes

4 ounces feta cheese with sun-dried tomatoes and basil

1. Bring water to boil in large saucepan over medium-high heat. Add lentils; cook 12 minutes.

2. Add orzo; cook 10 minutes or just until tender. Drain and rinse under cold water to cool completely. Drain well.

3. Meanwhile, combine tomatoes, celery, onion, olives, vinegar, oil, basil, garlic and red pepper flakes in large bowl; mix well.

4. Add lentil mixture to tomato mixture; toss gently to blend. Add cheese; toss gently. Let stand 15 minutes before serving.

MAKES 4 SERVINGS

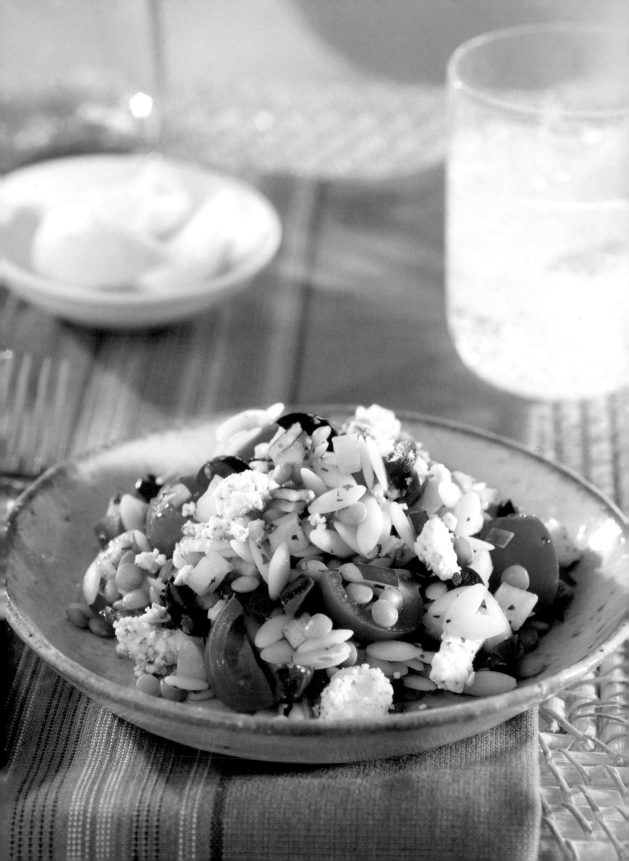

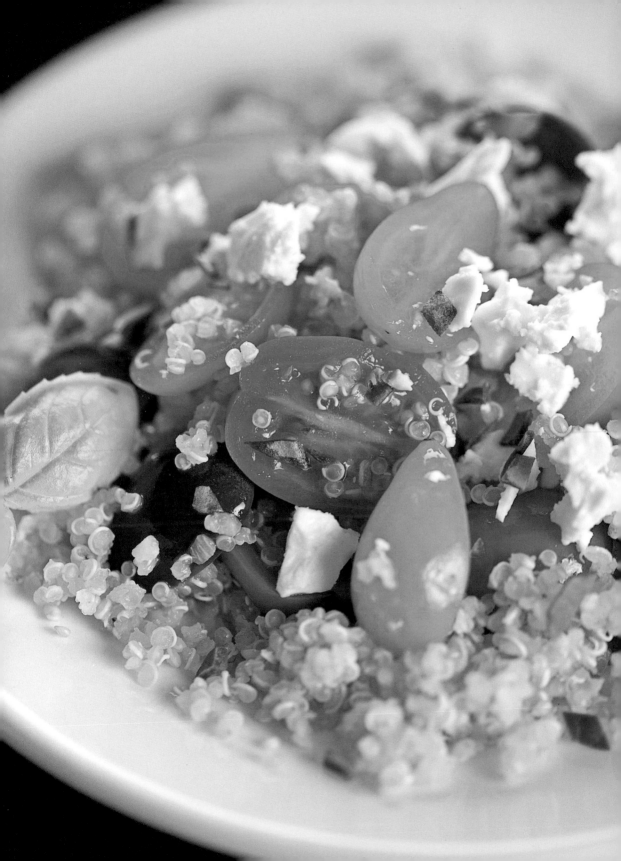

HEIRLOOM TOMATO QUINOA SALAD

1 cup uncooked quinoa

2 cups water

2 tablespoons olive oil

1 tablespoon lemon juice

1 clove garlic, minced

½ teaspoon salt

2 cups assorted heirloom grape tomatoes (red, yellow or a combination), halved

¼ cup crumbled feta cheese

¼ cup chopped fresh basil, plus additional basil leaves for garnish

1. Place quinoa in fine-mesh strainer; rinse well under cold water. Bring 2 cups water to a boil in small saucepan over medium-high heat; stir in quinoa. Reduce heat to low; cover and simmer 10 to 15 minutes or until quinoa is tender and water is absorbed.

2. Meanwhile, whisk oil, lemon juice, garlic and salt in large bowl until well blended. Gently stir in tomatoes and quinoa. Cover and refrigerate at least 30 minutes.

3. Stir in cheese just before serving. Top with chopped basil; garnish with additional basil leaves.

MAKES 4 SERVINGS

SHRIMP AND SOBA NOODLE SALAD

4 ounces soba noodles, cooked and well drained

1 package (12 ounces) medium shrimp, cooked, peeled and drained*

2 cups coarsely chopped broccoli florets, cooked until crisp-tender and drained

¼ cup minced green onions

2 tablespoons reduced-sodium soy sauce

2 tablespoons garlic-chili sauce**

1 tablespoon sesame or canola oil

½ teaspoon grated fresh ginger

1 tablespoon toasted sesame seeds (optional)

*Or use 1 package (12 ounces) frozen peeled cooked baby shrimp. Drain well, squeezing out excess moisture before adding to salad.

**Garlic-chili sauce can be found in the Asian section of most supermarkets and in Asian specialty markets.

1. Combine noodles, shrimp, broccoli and green onions in large serving bowl.

2. Combine soy sauce, garlic-chili sauce, oil and ginger in small bowl; mix well. Pour over noodle mixture; toss gently to coat. Let stand 10 minutes for flavors to blend. Garnish with sesame seeds, if desired.

MAKES 2 SERVINGS

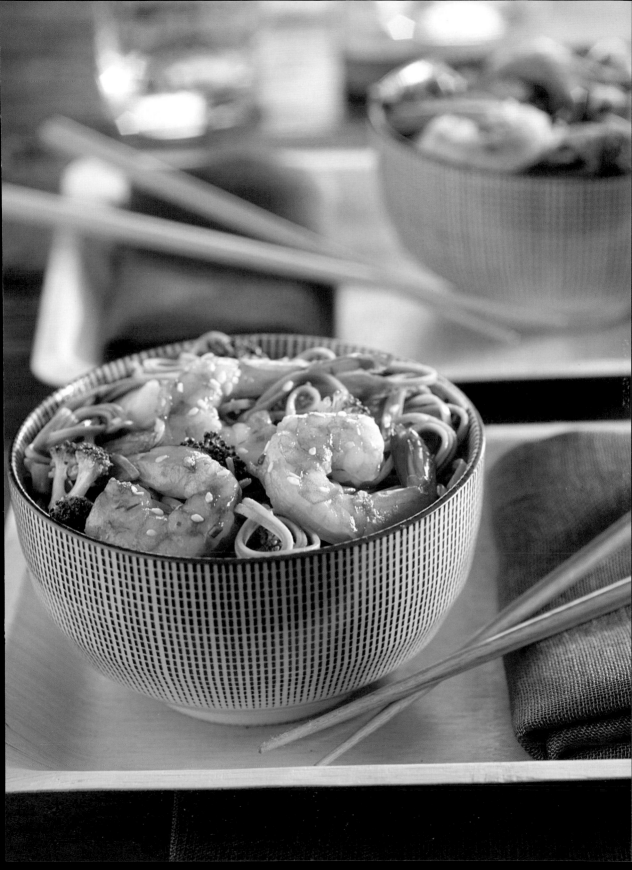

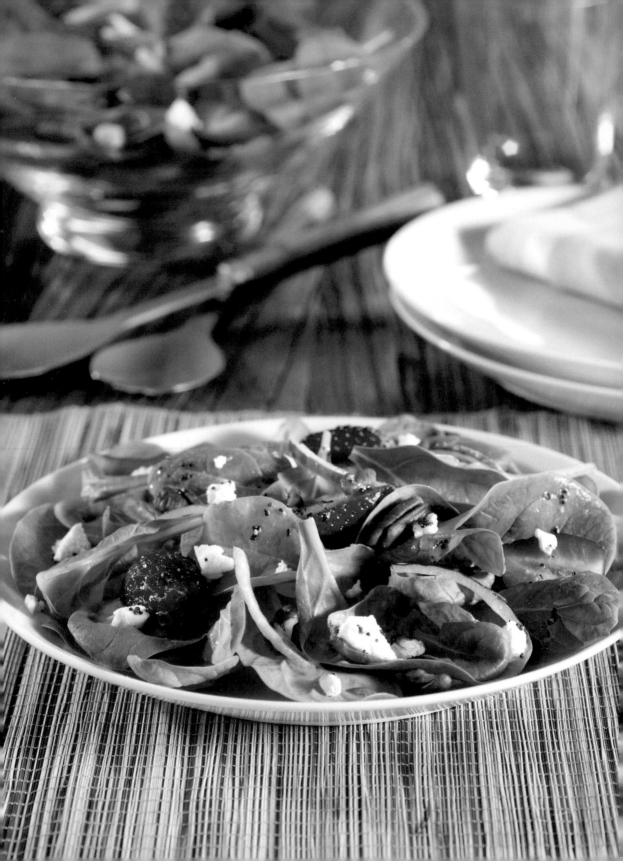

STRAWBERRY SPINACH SALAD WITH POPPY SEED DRESSING

6 cups baby spinach

8 fresh strawberries, halved

¼ cup chopped pecans, toasted*

¼ cup thinly sliced red onion

2 ounces goat cheese, crumbled

2 tablespoons canola oil

2 tablespoons unseasoned rice vinegar or raspberry vinegar

2 teaspoons honey

1 teaspoon ground dry mustard

Black pepper

½ teaspoon poppy seeds

*To toast pecans, cook in medium skillet over medium heat 1 to 2 minutes or until lightly browned, stirring frequently.

1. Place 1½ cups spinach on each of 4 plates. Top with strawberries, pecans, onion and cheese.

2. Whisk oil, vinegar, honey, mustard, pepper and poppy seeds in small bowl until blended. Drizzle dressing over salads.

MAKES 4 SERVINGS

CHICKEN AND PASTA SALAD WITH KALAMATA OLIVES

4 ounces uncooked multigrain rotini pasta

2 cups diced cooked chicken

½ cup chopped roasted red bell peppers

12 pitted kalamata olives, halved

2 tablespoons extra virgin olive oil

1 tablespoon dried basil

1 tablespoon cider vinegar

1 clove garlic, minced

¼ teaspoon salt

1. Cook pasta according to package directions; drain well. Set aside to cool.

2. Combine chicken, bell peppers, olives, oil, basil, vinegar, garlic and salt in large bowl; toss to coat.

3. Add cooled pasta to chicken mixture; toss gently.

MAKES 4 SERVINGS

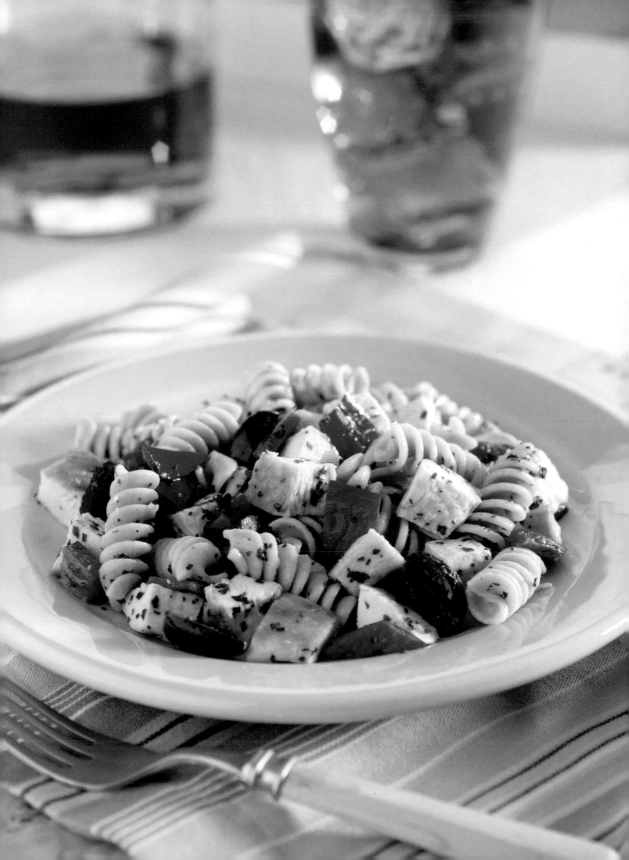

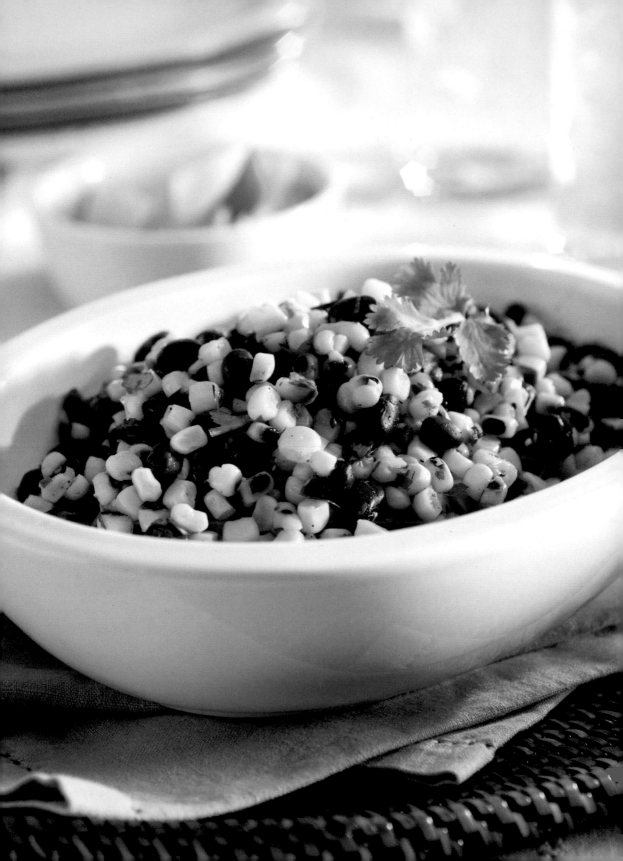

CHARRED CORN SALAD

3 tablespoons fresh lime juice

½ teaspoon salt

¼ cup extra virgin olive oil

4 to 6 ears corn, husked (enough to make 3 to 4 cups kernels)

⅔ cup canned black beans, rinsed and drained

½ cup chopped fresh cilantro

2 teaspoons minced seeded chipotle pepper (1 canned chipotle pepper in adobo sauce *or* 1 dried chipotle pepper, reconstituted in boiling water)*

*Chipotle peppers can sting and irritate the skin, so wear rubber gloves when handling peppers and do not touch your eyes.

1. Whisk lime juice and salt in small bowl. Gradually whisk in oil until blended.

2. Heat large skillet over medium-high heat. Cook corn in single layer 15 to 17 minutes or until browned and tender, turning frequently. Transfer to plate to cool slightly. Place in medium bowl.

3. Place beans in small microwavable bowl; microwave on HIGH 1 minute or until heated through. Add beans, cilantro and chipotle pepper to corn; mix well. Pour lime juice mixture over corn mixture; toss to coat.

MAKES 6 SERVINGS

Note: Since only a small amount of chipotle pepper is needed for this dish, store the leftovers into an airtight container and refrigerate or freeze.

MARKET SALAD

3 eggs

4 cups mixed baby salad greens

2 cups green beans, cut into 1½-inch pieces, cooked and drained

4 thick slices bacon, crisp-cooked and crumbled

1 tablespoon minced fresh basil, chives or Italian parsley

3 tablespoons olive oil

1 tablespoon red wine vinegar

1 teaspoon Dijon mustard

¼ teaspoon salt

¼ teaspoon black pepper

1. Place eggs in small saucepan; add water to cover. Bring to a boil over medium-high heat. Immediately remove from heat; cover and let stand 10 minutes. Drain and cool eggs to room temperature.

2. Combine salad greens, green beans, bacon and basil in large serving bowl. Peel and coarsely chop eggs; add to serving bowl.

3. Whisk oil, vinegar, mustard, salt and pepper in small bowl until well blended. Drizzle dressing over salad; toss gently to coat.

MAKES 4 SERVINGS

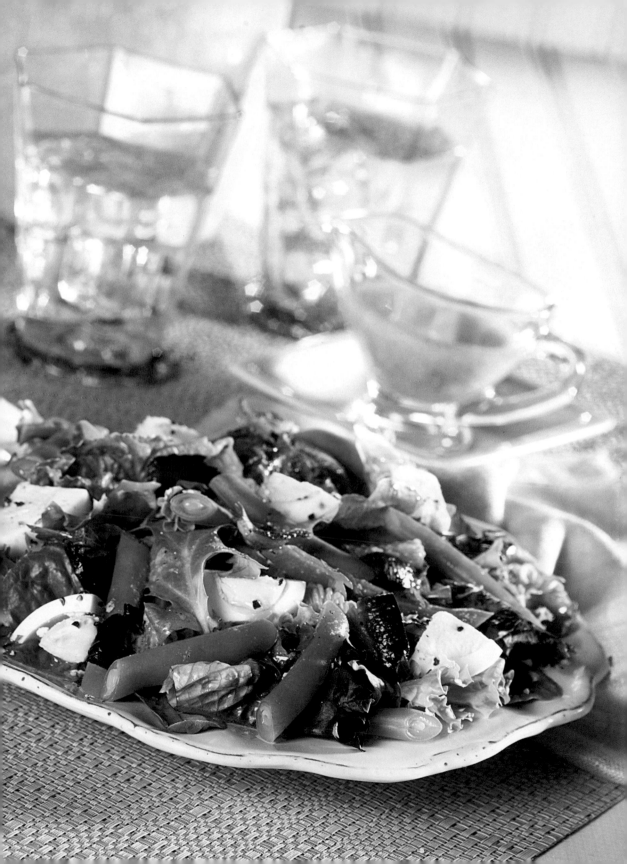

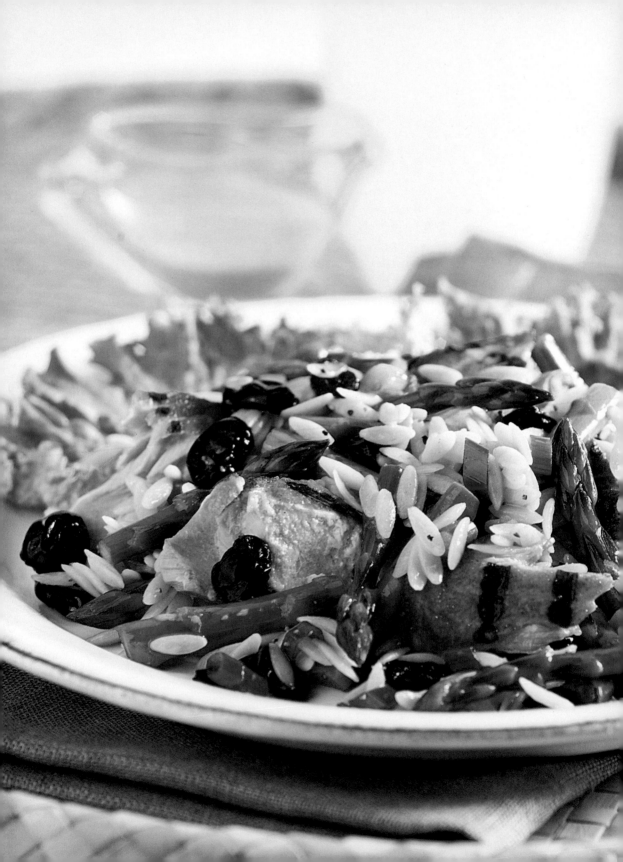

SALMON, ASPARAGUS AND ORZO SALAD

1 (8-ounce) salmon fillet

1 cup uncooked orzo pasta

8 ounces asparagus, cooked and cut into 2-inch pieces (about 1½ cups)

½ cup dried cranberries

¼ cup sliced green onions

3 tablespoons extra virgin olive oil

1 tablespoon white wine vinegar

1½ teaspoons Dijon mustard

½ teaspoon salt

⅛ teaspoon black pepper

1. Prepare grill for direct cooking. Oil grid.

2. Grill salmon over medium heat about 10 minutes per inch of thickness or until opaque in center. Remove to plate; cool 10 minutes. Flake salmon into bite-size pieces.

3. Meanwhile, cook orzo according to package directions; drain and cool.

4. Combine salmon, orzo, asparagus, cranberries and green onions in large bowl. Whisk oil, vinegar, mustard, salt and pepper in small bowl until well blended. Pour over salmon mixture; toss gently to coat. Refrigerate 30 minutes to 1 hour.

MAKES 4 TO 6 SERVINGS

VEGGIE SALAD WITH WHITE BEANS AND FETA

1 can (about 15 ounces) navy beans, rinsed and drained

1 can (14 ounces) quartered artichoke hearts, drained

1 green bell pepper, chopped

1 yellow bell pepper, chopped

1 cup grape tomatoes, halved

¼ cup chopped fresh basil *or* 1½ tablespoons dried basil plus ¼ cup chopped fresh parsley

¼ cup extra virgin olive oil

3 to 4 tablespoons red wine vinegar

1 teaspoon Dijon mustard

1 clove garlic, minced

½ teaspoon black pepper

¼ teaspoon salt

4 ounces crumbled feta cheese with sun-dried tomatoes and basil

1 package (about 5 ounces) spring greens mix

1. Combine beans, artichokes, bell peppers, tomatoes, basil, oil, vinegar, mustard, garlic, black pepper and salt in large bowl; toss gently to coat. Fold in cheese; let stand 10 minutes.

2. Place greens on 4 serving plates; top with vegetable mixture.

MAKES 4 SERVINGS

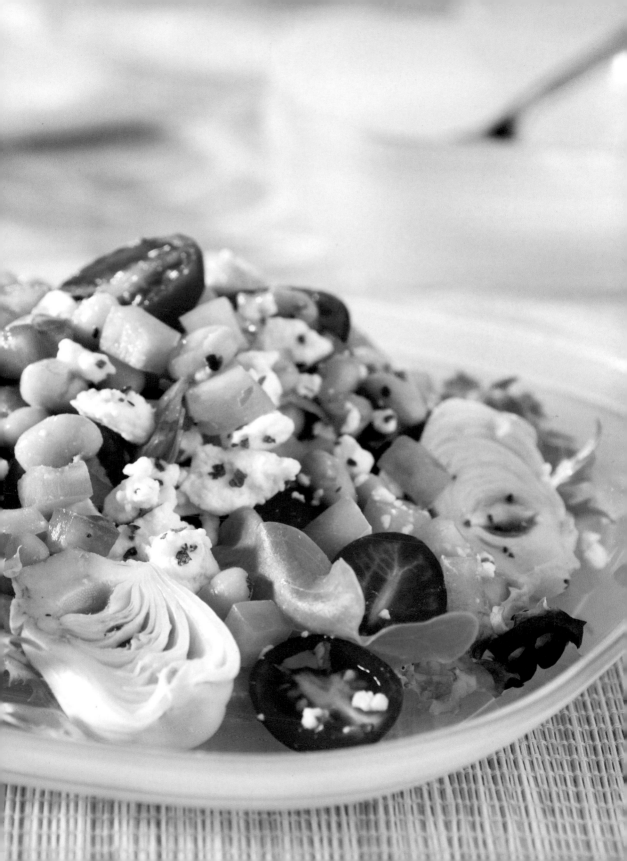

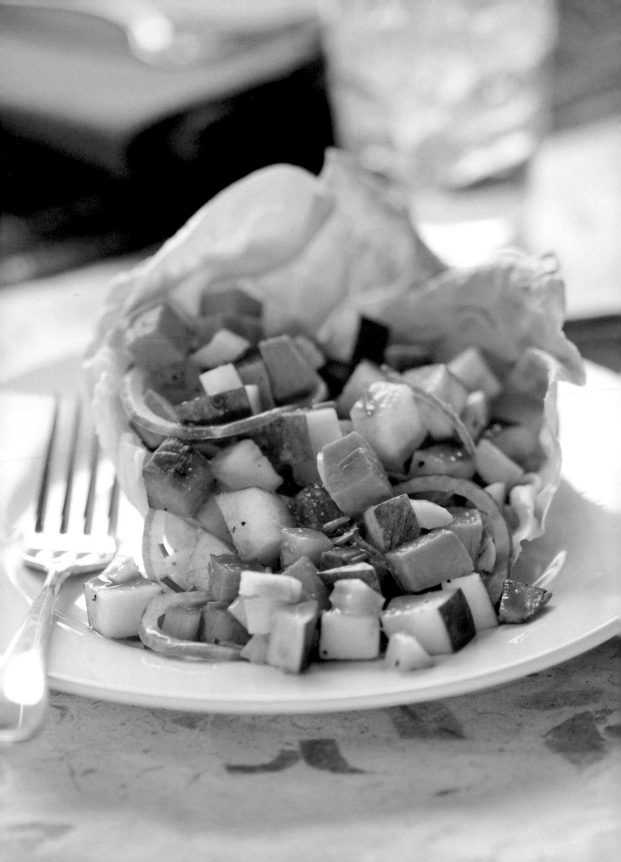

ROASTED SWEET POTATO AND APPLE SALAD

2 large sweet potatoes, peeled and cubed

2 tablespoons olive oil, divided

½ teaspoon salt, divided

¼ teaspoon black pepper

3 tablespoons apple juice

1 tablespoon balsamic vinegar

1 tablespoon Dijon mustard

1 tablespoon honey

2 teaspoons snipped fresh chives

1 medium Gala apple, diced (about 1 cup)

½ cup finely chopped celery

¼ cup thinly sliced red onion

Lettuce leaves

1. Preheat oven to 450°F. Spray baking sheet with nonstick cooking spray.

2. Combine sweet potatoes, 1 tablespoon oil, ¼ teaspoon salt and pepper on prepared baking sheet; toss to coat. Spread sweet potatoes in single layer.

3. Roast 20 to 25 minutes or until sweet potatoes are tender, stirring halfway through cooking time. Cool completely.

4. Meanwhile, whisk apple juice, remaining 1 tablespoon oil, vinegar, mustard, honey, chives and remaining ¼ teaspoon salt in small bowl until well blended.

5. Combine sweet potatoes, apple, celery and onion in medium bowl. Drizzle with dressing; gently toss to coat. Serve salad over lettuce leaves.

MAKES 4 SERVINGS

CHICKEN, PEACH AND CABBAGE SALAD

1½ cups diced cooked chicken breast, chilled

1 cup shredded red cabbage

1 medium ripe peach, peeled, pitted and cut into 1-inch pieces *or* 1 small mango, peeled and diced

1 stalk celery, diced

¼ cup plain yogurt

3 tablespoons peach nectar or orange juice

¼ teaspoon salt

¼ teaspoon curry powder

⅛ teaspoon black pepper

1. Combine chicken, cabbage, peach and celery in medium bowl; mix gently.

2. Whisk yogurt, peach nectar, salt, curry powder and pepper in small bowl until well blended. Add to chicken mixture; toss gently to coat.

MAKES 2 TO 3 SERVINGS

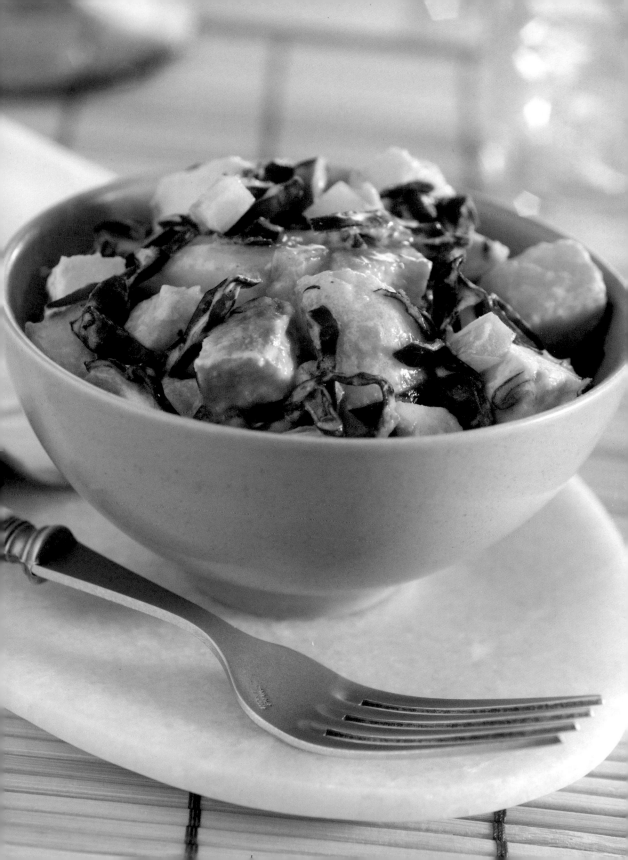

SOUPS

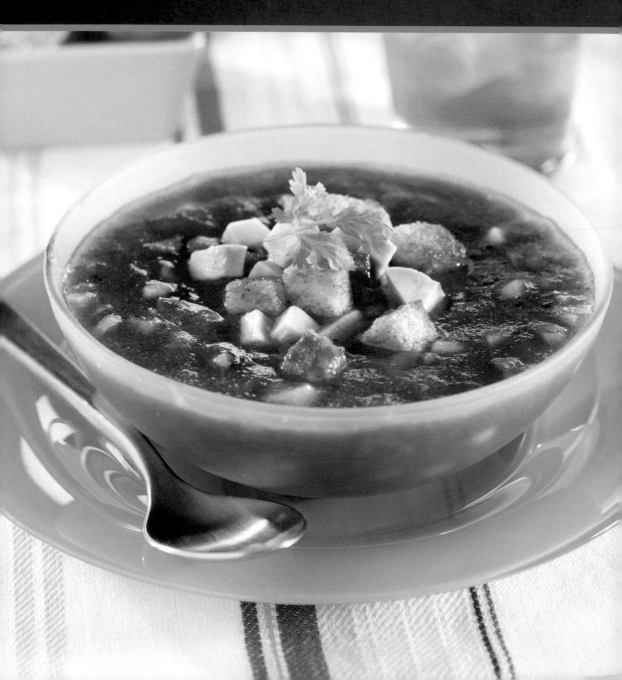

GAZPACHO

6 large, very ripe tomatoes (about 3 pounds), divided

1½ cups tomato juice

1 clove garlic

2 tablespoons lime juice

2 tablespoons olive oil

1 tablespoon white wine vinegar

1 teaspoon sugar

¾ teaspoon salt

½ teaspoon dried oregano

6 green onions, sliced

¼ cup finely chopped celery

¼ cup finely chopped seeded cucumber

1 or 2 fresh jalapeño peppers,* seeded, minced

Croutons (optional)

1 cup diced avocado

1 red or green bell pepper, chopped

2 tablespoons chopped fresh cilantro

Lime wedges (optional)

*Jalapeño peppers can sting and irritate the skin, so wear rubber gloves when handling peppers and do not touch your eyes.

1. Seed and finely chop 1 tomato; set aside.

2. Coarsely chop remaining 5 tomatoes. Combine half of tomatoes, ¾ cup tomato juice and garlic in food processor or blender; process until smooth. Press through sieve into large bowl; discard seeds. Repeat with remaining coarsely chopped tomatoes and ¾ cup tomato juice.

3. Whisk lime juice, oil, vinegar, sugar, salt and oregano into tomato mixture. Stir in finely chopped tomato, green onions, celery, cucumber and jalapeño pepper. Cover and refrigerate at least 4 hours or up to 24 hours to develop flavors.

4. Stir soup; ladle into chilled bowls. Top with croutons, if desired, avocado, bell pepper and cilantro. Serve with lime wedges, if desired.

MAKES 4 SERVINGS

CLASSIC LENTIL SOUP

3 tablespoons olive oil

1 medium onion, chopped

1 carrot, chopped

1 stalk celery, chopped

1 clove garlic, minced

8 ounces dried lentils, rinsed
   and sorted

3 cups chicken broth

1 can (about 14 ounces)
   stewed tomatoes

Salt and black pepper

½ cup grated Parmesan cheese
   (optional)

1. Heat oil in large skillet over medium heat. Add onion, carrot, celery and garlic; cook about 9 minutes or until vegetables are tender but not browned, stirring occasionally.

2. Stir in lentils, broth and tomatoes; bring to a boil over high heat. Reduce heat to low; cover and simmer 30 minutes or lentils are until tender.

3. Season with salt and pepper; sprinkle with cheese, if desired.

MAKES 4 TO 6 SERVINGS

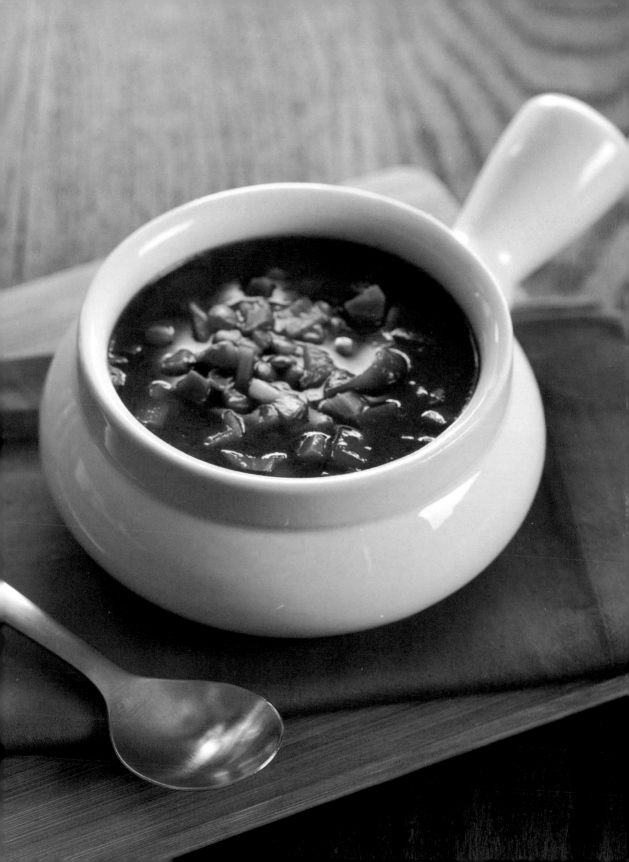

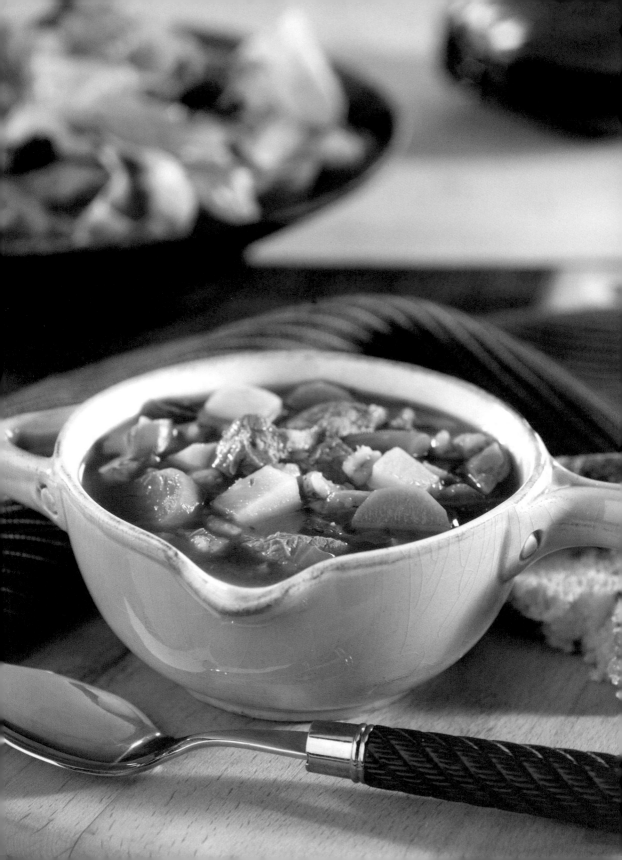

BEEF BARLEY SOUP

1 tablespoon olive oil

12 ounces boneless beef top round steak, trimmed and cut into ½-inch pieces

3 cans (about 14 ounces each) reduced-sodium beef broth

2 cups cubed unpeeled potatoes

1 can (about 14 ounces) diced tomatoes

1 cup chopped onion

1 cup sliced carrots

½ cup uncooked pearl barley

1 tablespoon cider vinegar

2 teaspoons caraway seeds

2 teaspoons dried marjoram

2 teaspoons dried thyme

½ teaspoon salt

½ teaspoon black pepper

1½ cups sliced green beans (½-inch slices)

1. Heat oil in large saucepan over medium heat. Add beef; cook and stir until browned on all sides.

2. Stir in broth, potatoes, tomatoes, onion, carrots, barley, vinegar, caraway seeds, marjoram, thyme, salt and pepper; bring to a boil over high heat. Reduce heat to low; cover and simmer 1½ hours.

3. Stir in green beans; cook, uncovered, 30 minutes or until beef is fork-tender.

MAKES 4 SERVINGS

CUBAN-STYLE BLACK BEAN SOUP

1 tablespoon olive oil

1 small onion, chopped

1 cup thinly sliced carrots

2 jalapeño peppers,* seeded and minced

2 cloves garlic, minced

1 can (about 15 ounces) black beans, undrained

1 can (about 14 ounces) vegetable or chicken broth

¼ cup sour cream

¼ cup chopped fresh cilantro

4 lime wedges (optional)

*Jalapeño peppers can sting and irritate the skin, so wear rubber gloves when handling peppers and do not touch your eyes.

1. Heat oil in large saucepan over medium heat. Add onion, carrots, jalapeño peppers and garlic; cook and stir 5 minutes.

2. Add beans and broth; bring to a boil. Reduce heat to low; cover and simmer 15 to 20 minutes or until vegetables are very tender.

3. Ladle soup into bowls; serve with sour cream, cilantro and lime wedges, if desired.

MAKES 4 (1-CUP) SERVINGS

Note: If a smoother texture is desired, purée soup in a food processor or blender.

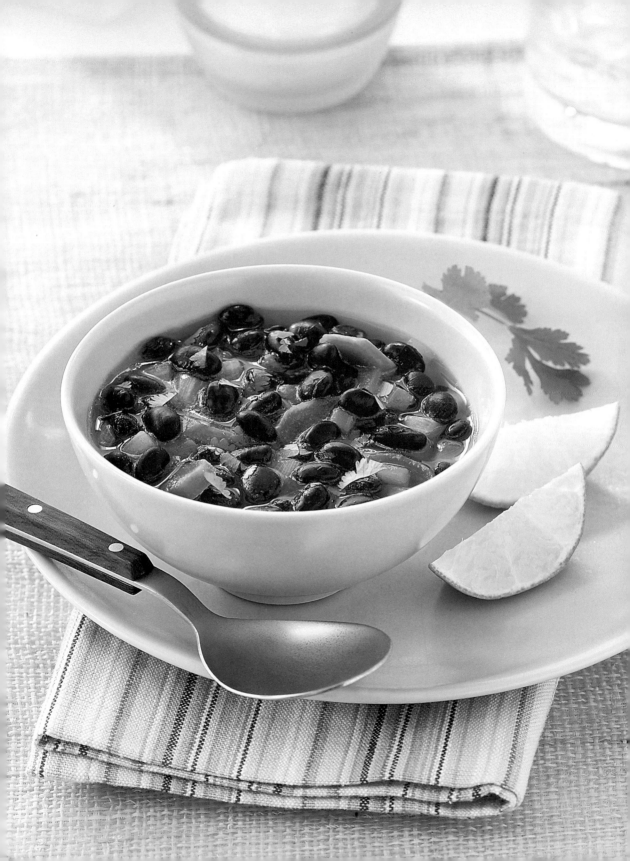

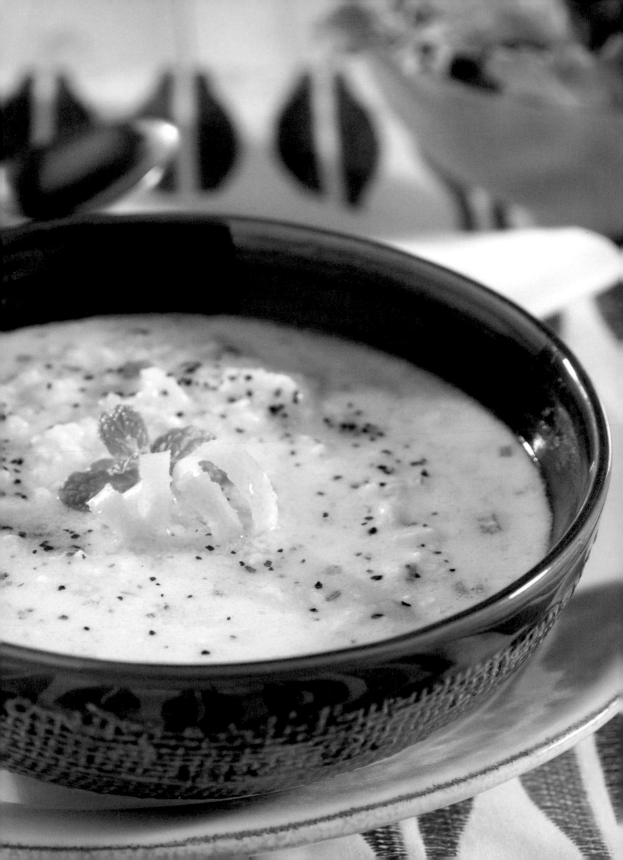

GREEK LEMON AND RICE SOUP

2 tablespoons butter

⅓ cup minced green onions

6 cups chicken broth

⅔ cup uncooked long grain rice

4 eggs

Juice of 1 lemon

⅛ teaspoon white pepper (optional)

Fresh mint leaves and lemon peel (optional)

1. Melt butter in medium saucepan over medium heat. Add green onions; cook and stir about 3 minutes or until tender.

2. Stir in broth and rice; bring to a boil over medium-high heat. Reduce heat to low; cover and simmer 20 to 25 minutes or until rice is tender.

3. Beat eggs in medium bowl. Stir in lemon juice and ½ cup hot broth mixture until blended. Gradually pour egg mixture back into broth mixture in saucepan, stirring constantly. Cook and stir over low heat 2 to 3 minutes or until soup thickens enough to lightly coat spoon. *Do not boil.*

4. Stir in pepper, if desired. Garnish with mint and lemon peel.

MAKES 6 TO 8 SERVINGS

SPICY SQUASH AND CHICKEN SOUP

1 tablespoon vegetable oil

1 small onion, finely chopped

1 stalk celery, finely chopped

2 cups cubed delicata or
    butternut squash
    (about 1 small)

2 cups chicken broth

1 can (about 14 ounces) diced
    tomatoes with green chiles

1 cup chopped cooked chicken

½ teaspoon salt

½ teaspoon ground ginger

⅛ teaspoon ground cumin

⅛ teaspoon black pepper

2 teaspoons lime juice

    Fresh parsley or cilantro sprigs
    (optional)

1. Heat oil in large saucepan over medium heat. Add onion and celery; cook and stir 5 minutes or just until tender.

2. Stir in squash, broth, tomatoes, chicken, salt, ginger, cumin and pepper; bring to a boil. Reduce heat to low; cover and cook 30 minutes or until squash is tender. Stir in lime juice. Garnish with parsley.

MAKES 4 SERVINGS

Tip: Delicata and butternut are two types of winter squash. Delicata is an elongated, creamy yellow squash with green striations. Butternut is a long, light orange squash. To use, cut the squash lengthwise, scoop out the seeds, peel and cut into cubes.

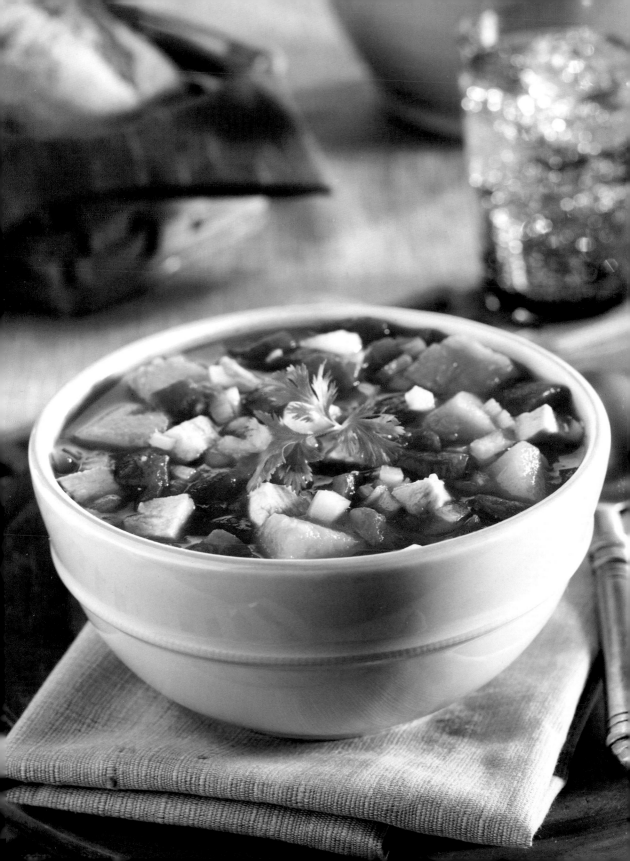

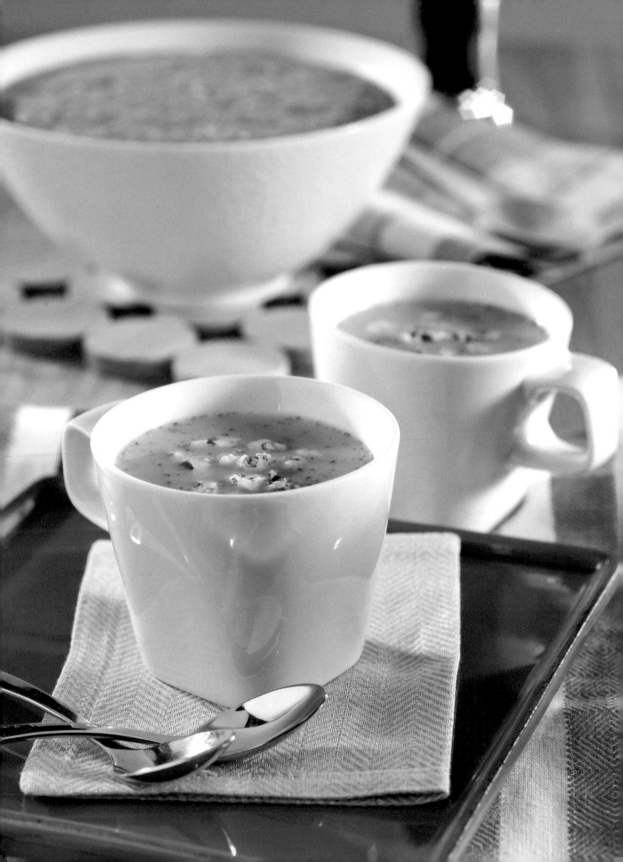

QUICK BROCCOLI SOUP

4 cups reduced-sodium chicken
   or vegetable broth

2½ pounds broccoli florets

1 onion, quartered

1 cup milk

¼ teaspoon salt

¼ cup crumbled blue cheese

1. Combine broth, broccoli and onion in large saucepan; bring to a boil over high heat. Reduce heat to low; cover and simmer about 20 minutes or until vegetables are tender.

2. Purée soup in blender and return to saucepan. Stir in milk and salt; cook until heated through.

3. Ladle soup into serving bowls; sprinkle with cheese.

MAKES 6 SERVINGS

TUSCAN WHITE BEAN SOUP

10 cups chicken broth

1 package (16 ounces) dried
   Great Northern beans,
   rinsed and sorted

1 can (about 14 ounces)
   diced tomatoes

1 large onion, chopped

3 carrots, chopped

6 ounces bacon, crisp-cooked
   and diced

4 cloves garlic, minced

1 sprig fresh rosemary *or*
   1 teaspoon dried rosemary

1 teaspoon black pepper

SLOW COOKER DIRECTIONS

1. Combine broth, beans, tomatoes, onion, carrots, bacon, garlic, rosemary and pepper to 5-quart slow cooker.

2. Cover; cook on LOW 8 hours. Remove and discard rosemary before serving.

MAKES 8 TO 10 SERVINGS

Serving Suggestion: Place slices of toasted Italian bread in individual soup bowls; drizzle with olive oil. Ladle soup over bread.

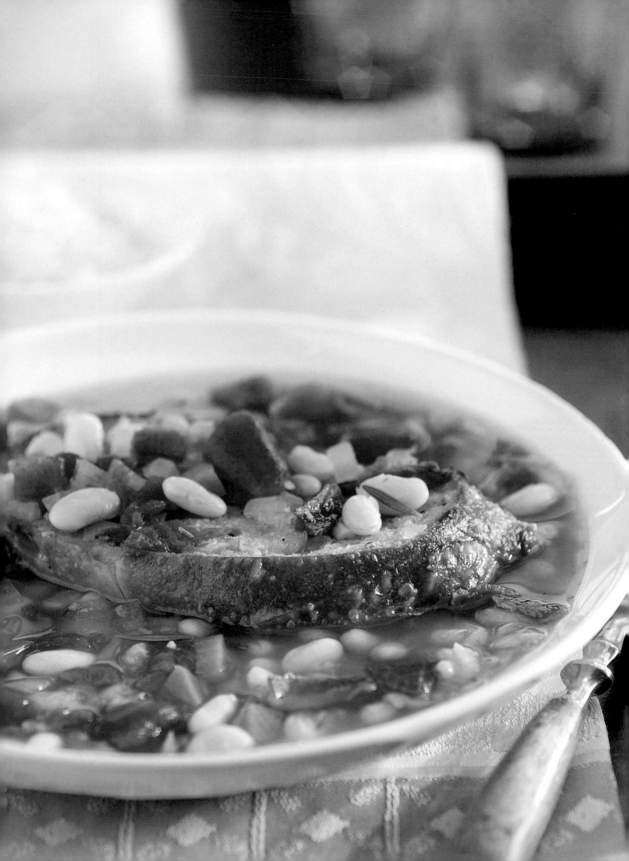

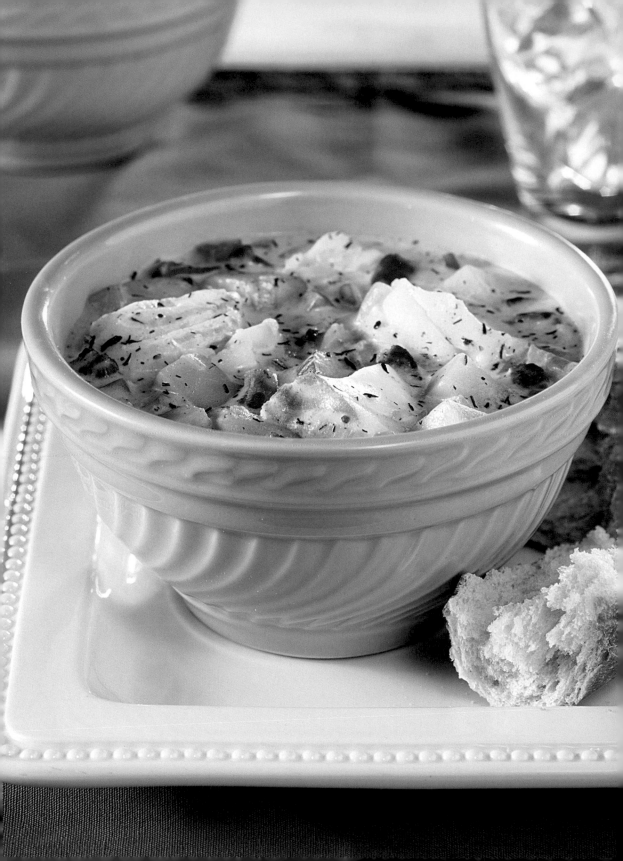

NEW ENGLAND FISH CHOWDER

4 ounces bacon, diced
1 cup chopped onion
½ cup chopped celery
2 cups diced peeled russet
   potatoes
2 tablespoons all-purpose flour
2 cups water
1 teaspoon salt

1 bay leaf
1 teaspoon dried dill weed
½ teaspoon dried thyme
½ teaspoon black pepper
1 pound cod, haddock or halibut
   fillets, skinned, boned and
   cut into 1-inch pieces
2 cups milk or half-and-half

1. Cook bacon in large saucepan over medium-high heat, stirring occasionally. Drain on paper towel-lined plate.

2. Add onion and celery to drippings in saucepan; cook and stir until onion is soft. Add potatoes; cook and stir 1 minute. Add flour; cook and stir 1 minute. Add water, salt, bay leaf, dill, thyme and pepper; bring to a boil over high heat. Reduce heat to low; cover and simmer 25 minutes or until potatoes are fork-tender.

3. Add fish to saucepan; cover and simmer 5 minutes or until fish begins to flake when tested with fork. Remove and discard bay leaf. Stir in bacon. Add milk; cook and stir until heated through. *Do not boil.*

MAKES 4 TO 6 SERVINGS

HOT AND SOUR SOUP WITH BOK CHOY AND TOFU

1 tablespoon dark sesame oil

4 ounces fresh shiitake mushrooms, stems finely chopped, caps thinly sliced

2 cloves garlic, minced

2 cups mushroom broth or vegetable broth

1 cup plus 2 tablespoons cold water, divided

2 tablespoons reduced-sodium soy sauce

1½ tablespoons rice vinegar or white wine vinegar

¼ teaspoon red pepper flakes

1½ tablespoons cornstarch

2 cups coarsely chopped bok choy leaves or napa cabbage

10 ounces silken extra firm tofu, well drained, cut into ½-inch cubes

1 green onion, thinly sliced

1. Heat oil in large saucepan over medium heat. Add mushrooms and garlic; cook and stir 4 minutes. Add broth, 1 cup water, soy sauce, vinegar and red pepper flakes; bring to a boil. Reduce heat to low; cook 5 minutes.

2. Whisk remaining 2 tablespoons water into cornstarch in small bowl until smooth. Stir into soup; cook 2 minutes or until thickened. Stir in bok choy; cook 2 to 3 minutes or until wilted. Stir in tofu; heat through. Sprinkle with green onion.

MAKES 4 SERVINGS

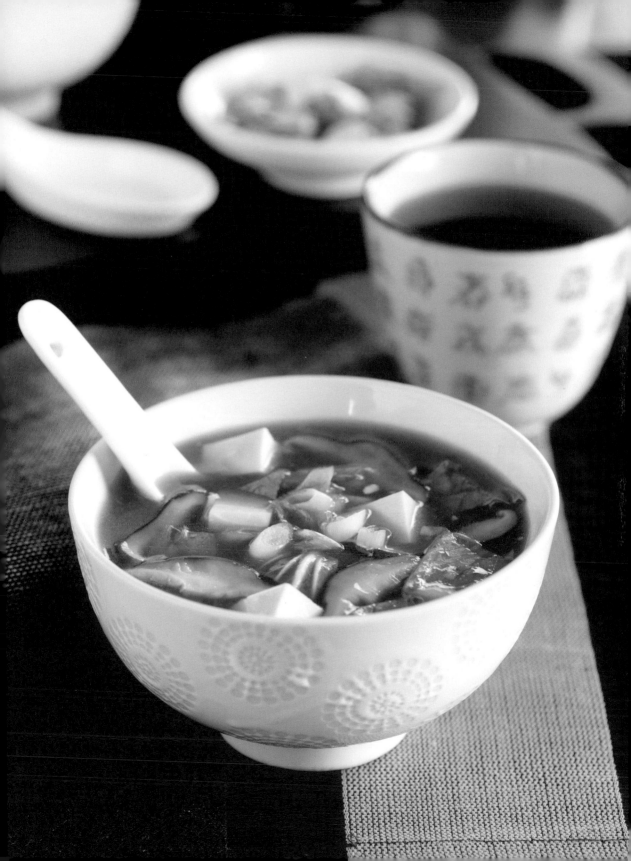

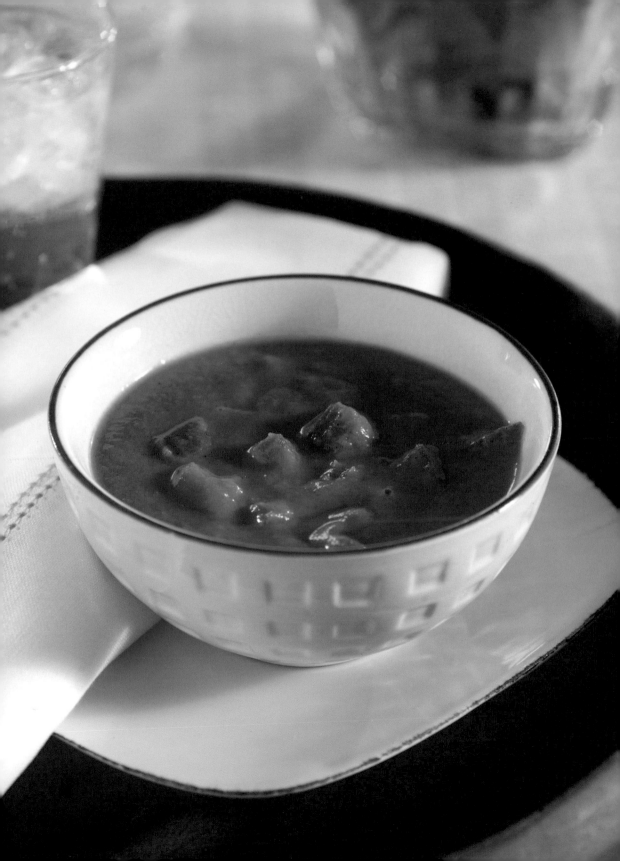

CHUNKY TOMATO-BASIL SOUP

2 tablespoons olive oil

1 cup chopped onion

2 cloves garlic, minced

5 cups fresh tomatoes, peeled, seeded and chopped, divided

1 can (6 ounces) tomato paste

1½ teaspoons dried basil

½ teaspoon salt

½ teaspoon dried marjoram

¼ teaspoon black pepper

4 cups reduced-sodium chicken broth

1. Heat oil in large saucepan over medium heat. Add onion and garlic; cover and cook 7 minutes or until onion is tender, stirring occasionally.

2. Reserve 1 cup fresh tomatoes. Add remaining tomatoes to saucepan. Stir in tomato paste, basil, salt, marjoram and pepper. Stir in broth; bring to a boil. Reduce heat to low; cover and simmer 30 minutes.

3. Working in batches, blend soup in blender* or food processor until smooth. Return puréed soup to saucepan. Stir in reserved tomatoes; cook until heated through.

*Or use hand held immersion blender.

MAKES 6 SERVINGS

MIDDLE EASTERN CHICKEN SOUP

1 can (about 14 ounces) reduced-sodium chicken broth

1 can (about 15 ounces) chickpeas, rinsed and drained

1 cup chopped cooked chicken

1 small onion, chopped

1 carrot, chopped

1 clove garlic, minced

1 teaspoon dried oregano

1 teaspoon ground cumin

½ (10-ounce) package fresh spinach, stemmed and coarsely chopped

⅛ teaspoon black pepper

1. Combine broth, 1½ cans water, chickpeas, chicken, onion, carrot, garlic, oregano and cumin in medium saucepan; bring to a boil over high heat. Reduce heat to medium-low; cover and simmer 15 minutes.

2. Stir in spinach and pepper; simmer, uncovered, 2 minutes or until spinach is wilted.

MAKES 4 SERVINGS

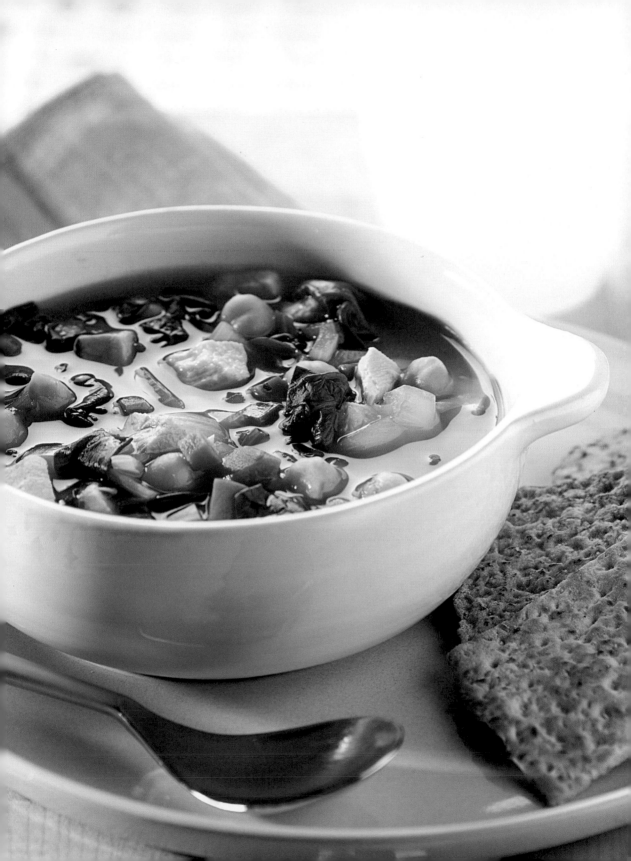

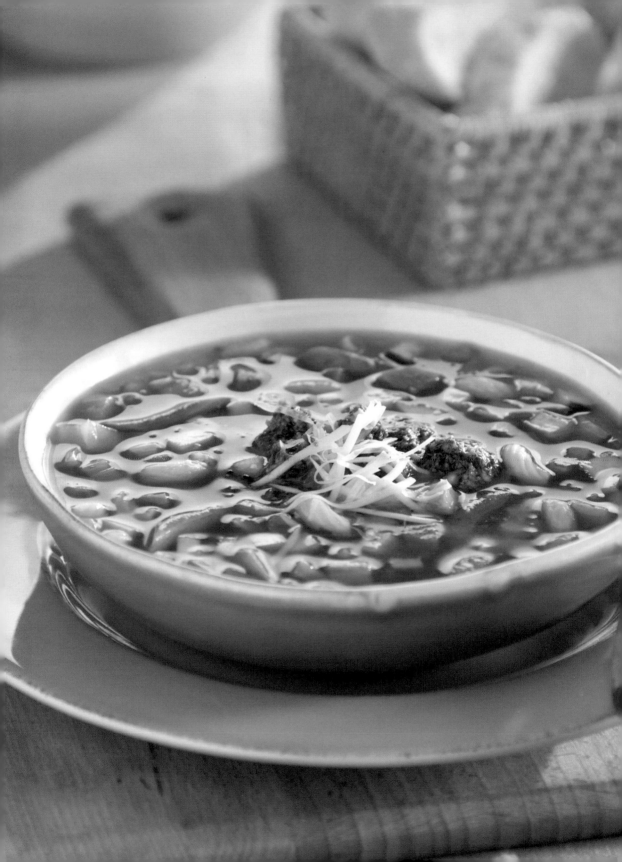

FRENCH PEASANT SOUP

1 slice bacon, chopped

½ cup diced carrots

½ cup diced celery

¼ cup minced onion

1 clove garlic, minced

2 tablespoons dry white wine or water

1 can (about 14 ounces) vegetable broth

1 sprig fresh thyme *or* 1 teaspoon dried thyme

1 bay leaf

1 sprig fresh parsley *or* 1 teaspoon dried parsley flakes

½ cup chopped green beans (½-inch pieces)

2 tablespoons uncooked small pasta or elbow macaroni

1 cup canned cannellini beans, drained and rinsed

½ cup diced zucchini

¼ cup chopped leek

2 teaspoons prepared pesto sauce

2 teaspoons grated Parmesan cheese

1. Cook bacon in medium saucepan over medium heat 3 minutes or until partially cooked. Add carrots, celery, onion and garlic; cook and stir 5 minutes or until carrots are crisp-tender. Stir in wine; cook until most of wine has evaporated. Add broth, thyme, bay leaf and parsley; cook 10 minutes.

2. Add green beans; cook 5 minutes. Add pasta; cook 5 to 7 minutes or until almost tender.

3. Add cannellini beans, zucchini and leek; cook 5 minutes or until vegetables are tender.

4. Remove and discard bay leaf. Ladle soup into 2 bowls. Stir 1 teaspoon pesto into each bowl; sprinkle with cheese.

MAKES 2 SERVINGS

ENTRÉES

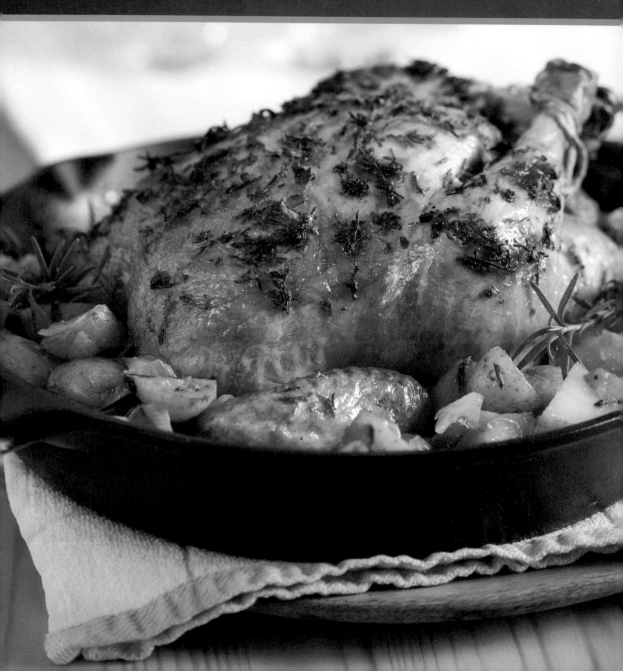

LEMON GARLIC ROAST CHICKEN

4 sprigs fresh rosemary, divided

6 cloves garlic, divided

1 lemon

2 tablespoons butter, softened

2 teaspoons salt, divided

2 large russet potatoes, cut into ¾-inch pieces

2 onions, cut into 1-inch pieces

2 tablespoons olive oil

½ teaspoon black pepper

1 whole chicken (3 to 4 pounds)

1. Preheat oven to 400°F. Finely chop 2 sprigs rosemary (about 2 tablespoons). Mince 3 cloves garlic. Grate peel from lemon. Combine butter, chopped rosemary, minced garlic, lemon peel and ½ teaspoon salt in small bowl; mix well. Set aside while preparing vegetables.

2. Combine potatoes, onions, oil, 1 teaspoon salt and pepper in medium bowl; toss to coat. Spread mixture in single layer in large (12-inch) cast iron skillet.

3. Smash remaining 3 cloves garlic. Cut lemon into quarters. Season cavity of chicken with remaining ½ teaspoon salt. Place garlic, lemon quarters and remaining 2 sprigs rosemary in cavity; tie legs with kitchen string, if desired. Place chicken on top of vegetables in skillet; spread butter mixture over chicken.

4. Roast about 1 hour or until chicken is cooked through (165°F) and potatoes are tender. Let stand 10 minutes before carving. Sprinkle with additional salt and pepper to taste.

MAKES 4 SERVINGS

SHRIMP AND VEGGIE SKILLET TOSS

¼ cup reduced-sodium soy sauce

2 tablespoons lime juice

1 tablespoon sesame oil

1 teaspoon grated fresh ginger

⅛ teaspoon red pepper flakes

2 teaspoons olive oil, divided

32 medium raw shrimp (about 8 ounces total), peeled and deveined (with tails on)

2 medium zucchini, each cut in half lengthwise, then cut crosswise into 6 pieces

6 green onions, trimmed and halved lengthwise

12 grape tomatoes

1. Whisk soy sauce, lime juice, sesame oil, ginger and red pepper flakes in small bowl until well blended.

2. Heat 1 teaspoon olive oil in large nonstick skillet over medium-high heat. Add shrimp; cook and stir 3 minutes or until shrimp are opaque. Remove to large bowl.

3. Heat remaining 1 teaspoon olive oil in same skillet. Add zucchini; cook and stir 4 to 6 minutes or just until crisp-tender. Add green onions and tomatoes; cook and stir 2 minutes. Add shrimp; cook 1 minute. Return to large bowl.

4. Add soy sauce mixture to skillet; bring to a boil. Pour over shrimp and vegetables; toss gently to coat.

MAKES 4 SERVINGS

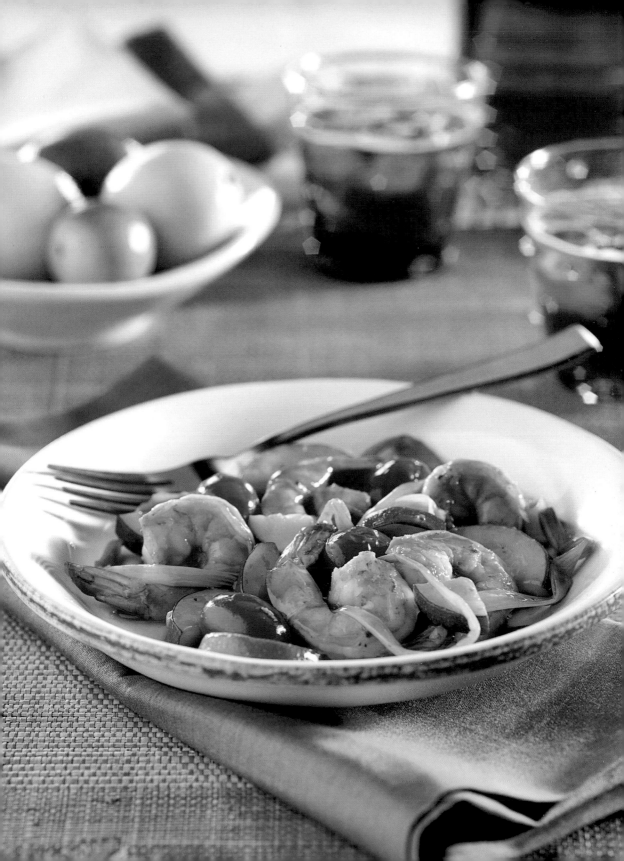

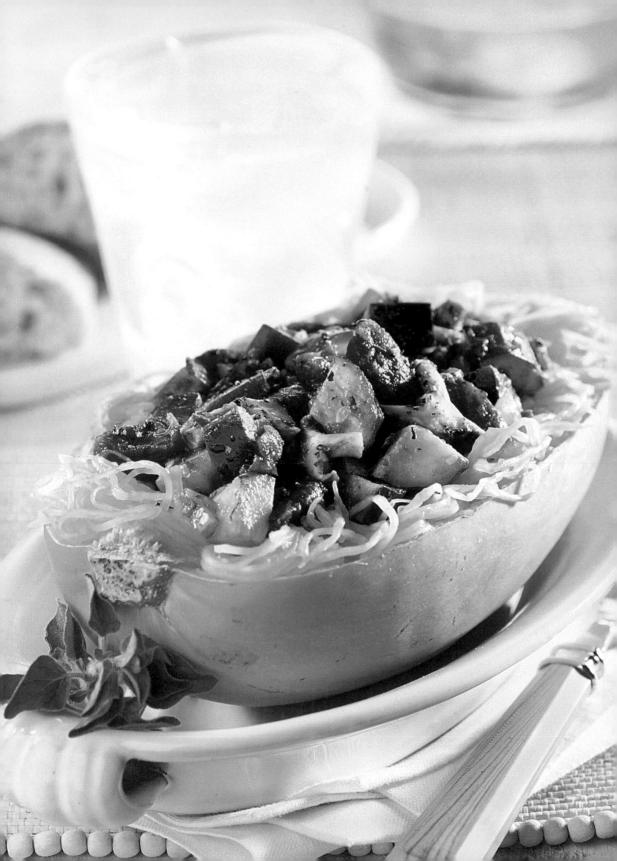

SPICY RATATOUILLE WITH SPAGHETTI SQUASH

1 spaghetti squash (2 pounds)
2 tablespoons olive oil
1 small onion, finely chopped
1 clove garlic, minced
1 small eggplant, diced
1 small zucchini, diced
1 cup coarsely chopped mushrooms, preferably oyster or shiitake

1 can (about 14 ounces) diced tomatoes
1 tablespoon canned chipotle pepper in adobo sauce, minced
½ teaspoon dried oregano
½ teaspoon salt
¼ teaspoon black pepper
Grated Parmesan cheese (optional)

1. Pierce squash skin with fork or paring knife several times; place on microwavable plate. Cover loosely with plastic wrap; microwave on HIGH 12 to 13 minutes, turning after 6 minutes. (Squash is fully cooked when fork pierces skin and flesh easily.) Set aside to cool 5 minutes.

2. When squash is cool enough to handle, cut in half lengthwise. Scoop out and discard seeds. Separate squash into strands with fork. Measure 2 cups; cover and set aside. Save the empty squash shell halves, if desired.*

3. While squash cooks, heat oil in large skillet. Add onion and garlic; cook and stir over medium-high heat 1 minute. Add eggplant, zucchini and mushrooms; cook and stir heat 5 minutes or until vegetables are lightly browned. Stir in tomatoes, chipotle pepper, oregano, salt and pepper; cook over medium heat 3 to 5 minutes or until slightly thickened and heated through.

4. Spread squash on serving plate; top with ratatouille. Sprinkle with cheese, if desired. Serve immediately.

*For a unique presentation, serve the ratatouille in the empty squash shell halves.

MAKES 4 SERVINGS

BEEF AND PEPPER KABOBS

8 ounces sirloin steak

2 teaspoons reduced-sodium
soy sauce

2 teaspoons red wine vinegar

1½ teaspoons Dijon mustard

1 teaspoon olive oil

1 clove garlic, minced

⅛ teaspoon black pepper

2 small bell peppers (green,
red, yellow, orange or
a combination)

4 large green onions, trimmed

1 tablespoon chicken or
vegetable broth

1. Cut steak into 16 (¼-inch) strips; place in medium bowl. Whisk soy sauce, vinegar, mustard, oil, garlic and black pepper in small bowl until well blended. Pour half of marinade over steak; toss to coat. Cover and refrigerate 2 to 3 hours, stirring occasionally. Cover and refrigerate remaining marinade until ready to cook.

2. Prepare grill for direct cooking. Cut each bell pepper into 12 pieces. Thread 6 bell pepper pieces onto each of 4 metal skewers; grill 5 to 7 minutes per side or until well browned and tender. Add green onions to grill; grill 3 to 5 minutes or until well browned on both sides. Stir broth into reserved marinade; brush bell peppers and green onions lightly with marinade once during grilling.

3. Thread 4 beef strips onto each of 4 metal skewers. Grill 2 minutes per side, brushing once with broth mixture.

4. To serve, place 1 beef skewer and 1 bell pepper skewer on each of 4 plates. Remove beef and bell peppers from skewers. Chop green onions; sprinkle over each serving.

MAKES 4 SERVINGS

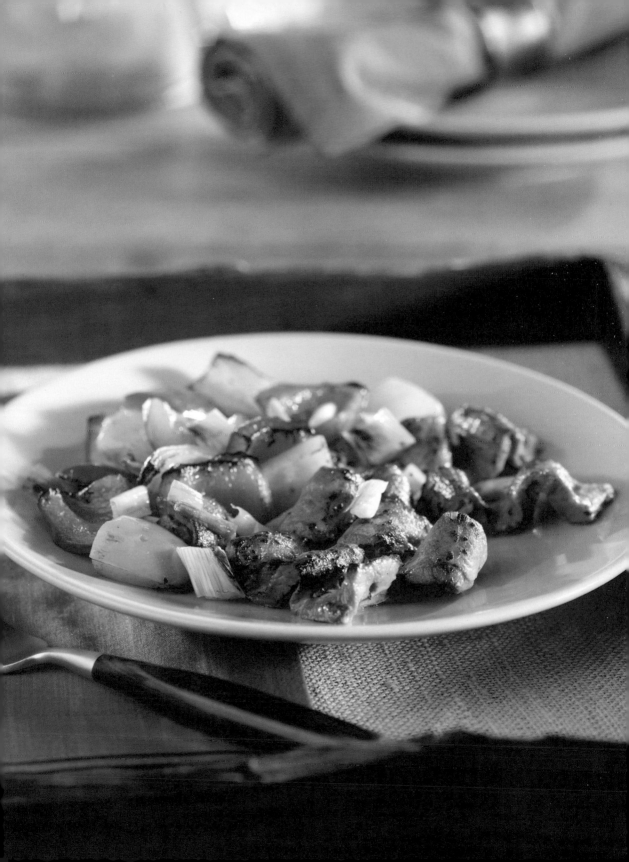

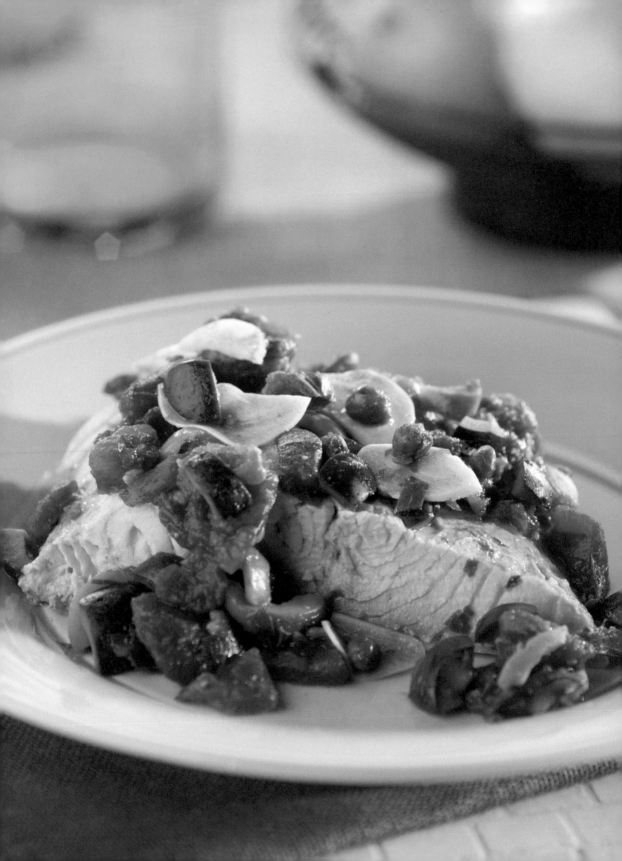

GREEK-STYLE SALMON

1 tablespoon olive oil

1¾ cups diced tomatoes, drained

6 pitted black olives, coarsely chopped

4 pitted green olives, coarsely chopped

3 tablespoons lemon juice

2 tablespoons chopped fresh Italian parsley

1 tablespoon capers, rinsed and drained

2 cloves garlic, thinly sliced

¼ teaspoon black pepper

1 pound salmon fillets

1. Heat oil in large skillet over medium heat. Add tomatoes, olives, lemon juice, parsley, capers, garlic and pepper; bring to a simmer, stirring frequently. Cook 5 minutes or until reduced by about one third, stirring occasionally.

2. Rinse salmon and pat dry with paper towels. Push sauce to one side of skillet. Add salmon; spoon sauce over salmon. Cover and cook 10 to 15 minutes or until salmon begins to flake when tested with fork.

MAKES 4 SERVINGS

SEARED SPICED PORK TENDERLOIN AND APPLES

½ teaspoon ground cinnamon

½ teaspoon ground cumin

½ teaspoon salt

½ teaspoon black pepper

⅛ teaspoon ground allspice

1 pound pork tenderloin

1 tablespoon olive oil

2 medium Fuji or Gala apples, sliced

¼ cup raisins

¼ cup water

1 tablespoon butter

1. Preheat oven to 425°F. Line baking sheet with foil. Combine cinnamon, cumin, salt, pepper and allspice in small bowl; mix well. Sprinkle evenly over all sides of pork, pressing to adhere.

2. Heat oil in large skillet over medium-high heat. Add pork; cook until browned on all sides, turning frequently. Transfer to prepared baking sheet.

3. Roast pork 18 minutes or until barely pink in center. Transfer to cutting board; let stand 5 minutes before cutting into thin slices.

4. Meanwhile, combine apples, raisins and water in same skillet; cook and stir over medium-high heat 2 minutes or until apples begin to brown. Remove from heat; stir in butter. Serve pork over apple mixture.

MAKES 4 SERVINGS

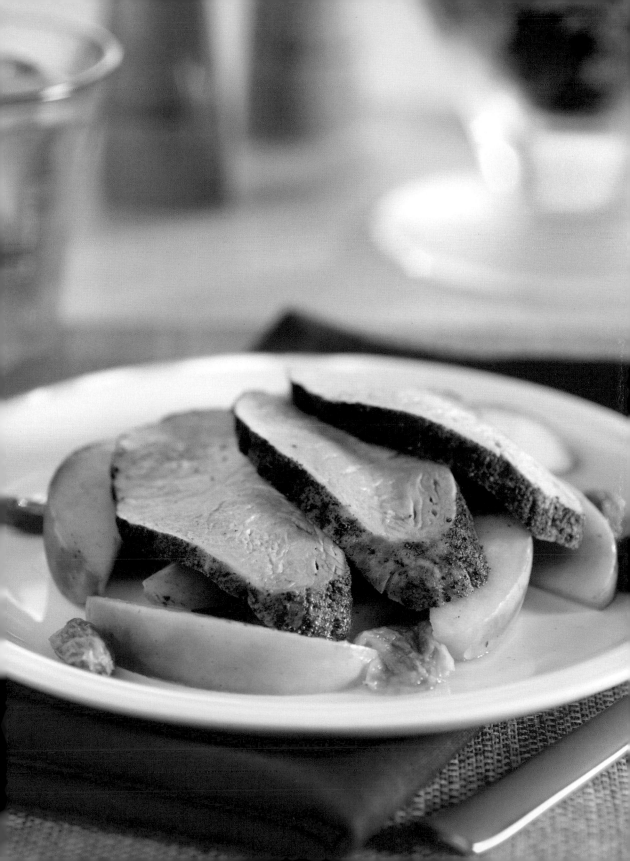

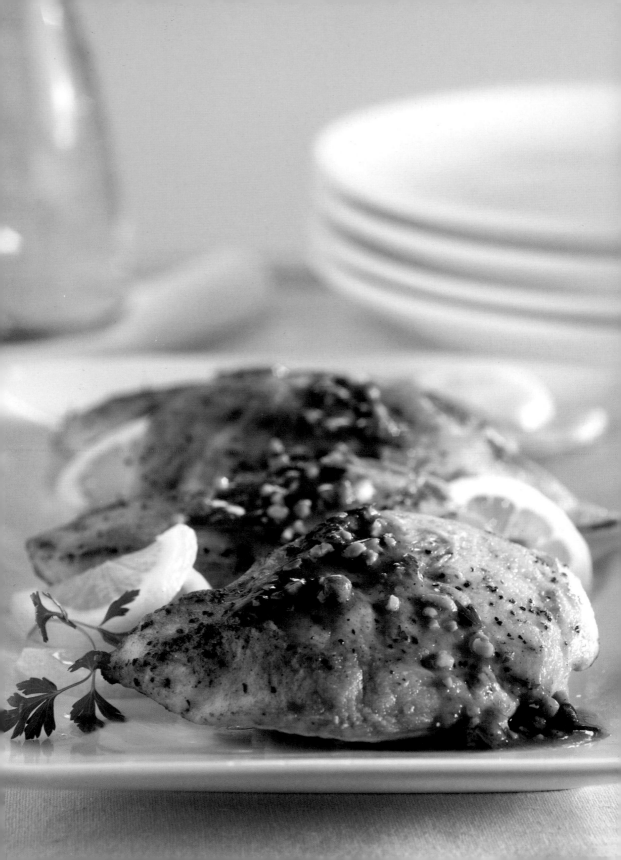

CHICKEN PICCATA

3 tablespoons all-purpose flour

½ teaspoon salt

¼ teaspoon black pepper

4 boneless skinless chicken breasts (4 ounces each)

2 teaspoons olive oil

1 teaspoon butter

2 cloves garlic, minced

¾ cup reduced-sodium chicken broth

1 tablespoon lemon juice

2 tablespoons chopped fresh Italian parsley

1 tablespoon capers, drained

1. Combine flour, salt and pepper in shallow dish. Reserve 1 tablespoon flour mixture; set aside.

2. Pound chicken to ½-inch thickness between sheets of waxed paper with flat side of meat mallet or rolling pin. Coat chicken with remaining flour mixture, shaking off excess.

3. Heat oil and butter in large nonstick skillet over medium heat. Add chicken; cook 4 to 5 minutes per side or until no longer pink in center. Transfer to serving platter; cover loosely with foil.

4. Add garlic to same skillet; cook and stir 1 minute. Add reserved 1 tablespoon flour mixture; cook and stir 1 minute. Add broth and lemon juice; cook 2 minutes or until thickened, stirring frequently. Stir in parsley and capers until blended. Spoon sauce over chicken.

MAKES 4 SERVINGS

TOFU, VEGETABLE AND CURRY STIR-FRY

1 package (about 14 ounces) extra-firm tofu, cut into ¾-inch cubes

¾ cup coconut milk

2 tablespoons lime juice

1 tablespoon curry powder

1 tablespoon dark sesame oil, divided

4 cups broccoli florets (1½-inch pieces)

2 medium red bell peppers, cut into short, thin strips

1 medium red onion, cut into thin wedges

¼ teaspoon salt

Hot cooked brown rice (optional)

1. Press tofu cubes between layers of paper towels to remove excess moisture. Combine coconut milk, lime juice and curry powder in medium bowl; mix well.

2. Heat 1 teaspoon oil in large nonstick skillet over medium heat. Add tofu; cook 10 minutes or until lightly browned on all sides, turning often. Remove to plate.

3. Add remaining 2 teaspoons oil to skillet. Add broccoli, bell pepper and onion; stir-fry over high heat about 5 minutes or until vegetables are crisp-tender. Add tofu and coconut milk mixture; cook and stir until mixture comes to a boil. Stir in salt. Serve immediately with rice, if desired.

MAKES 4 SERVINGS

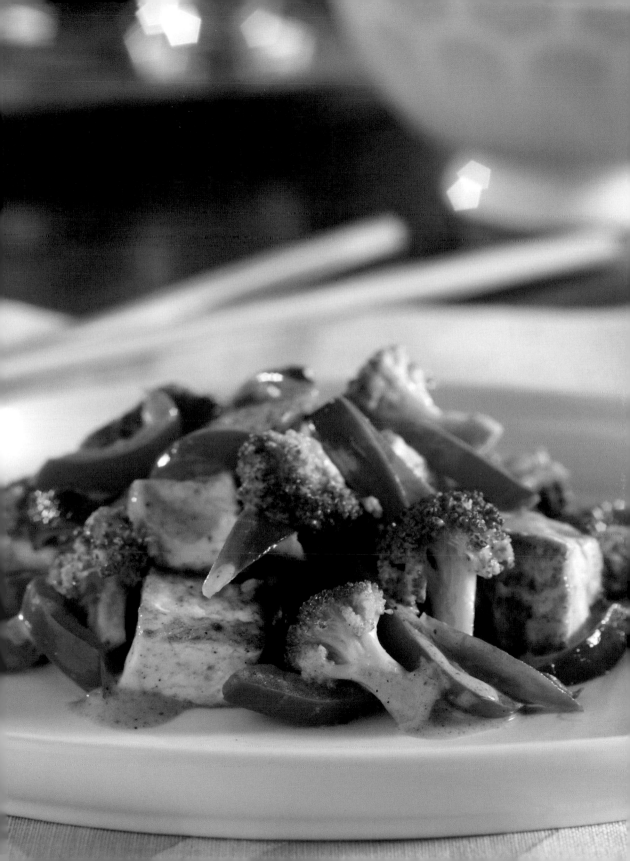

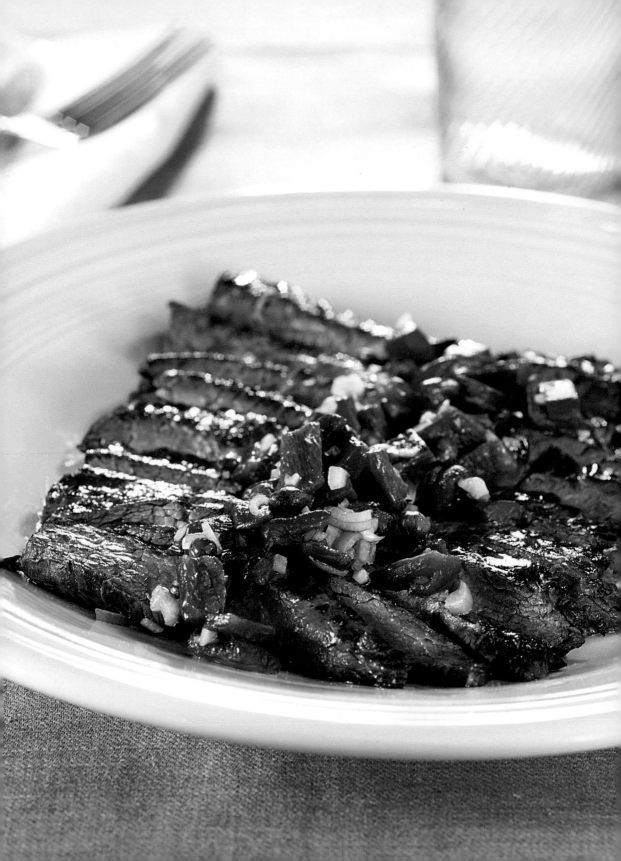

SKIRT STEAK WITH RED PEPPER CHIMICHURRI

1 pound skirt steak, trimmed

1 clove garlic, peeled and halved

¼ teaspoon salt

½ teaspoon black pepper, divided

1 cup diced roasted red pepper

1½ tablespoons olive oil

1 tablespoon white wine vinegar

1 shallot, minced

1 tablespoon capers, rinsed and drained

1 clove garlic, minced

1. Preheat broiler. Spray broiler rack with nonstick cooking spray. Rub steak on both sides with garlic clove. Season with salt and ¼ teaspoon black pepper. Place steak on broiler rack.

2. Broil steak 4 inches from heat 4 to 5 minutes per side or until desired doneness. Tent with foil; let stand 10 minutes before slicing.

3. Combine roasted pepper, oil, vinegar, shallot, capers, minced garlic and remaining ¼ teaspoon black pepper in medium bowl; mix well.

4. Thinly slice skirt steak against the grain; arrange on serving platter. Top with chimichurri sauce or serve sauce separately.

MAKES 4 SERVINGS

SHRIMP AND VEGETABLE SOUVLAKI

8 ounces raw shrimp, peeled
and deveined (with tails on)

1 medium zucchini, halved
lengthwise and cut into
½-inch slices

½ medium red bell pepper,
cut into 1-inch squares

8 green onions, trimmed
and cut into 2-inch pieces

2½ tablespoons extra virgin
olive oil, divided

2 tablespoons lemon juice

2 teaspoons grated lemon peel

2 cloves garlic, minced

½ teaspoon salt

½ teaspoon finely chopped
fresh rosemary

⅛ teaspoon red pepper flakes

1. Spray 4 (12-inch) bamboo or metal skewers with nonstick cooking spray. Alternately thread shrimp, zucchini, bell pepper and green onions onto skewers.

2. Whisk 2 tablespoons oil, lemon juice, lemon peel, garlic, salt, rosemary and red pepper flakes in small bowl until well blended.

3. Prepare grill for direct cooking. Spray grill rack or grill pan with nonstick cooking spray. Brush skewers lightly with remaining ½ tablespoon oil.

4. Grill skewers 2 minutes per side. Remove to serving platter; drizzle with sauce.

MAKES 4 SERVINGS

Note: "Souvlaki" is the Greek word for shishkebab. Souvlaki traditionally consists of fish or meat that has been seasoned in a mixture of oil, lemon juice and seasonings. Many souvlaki recipes, including this one, also include chunks of vegetables such as bell pepper and onion.

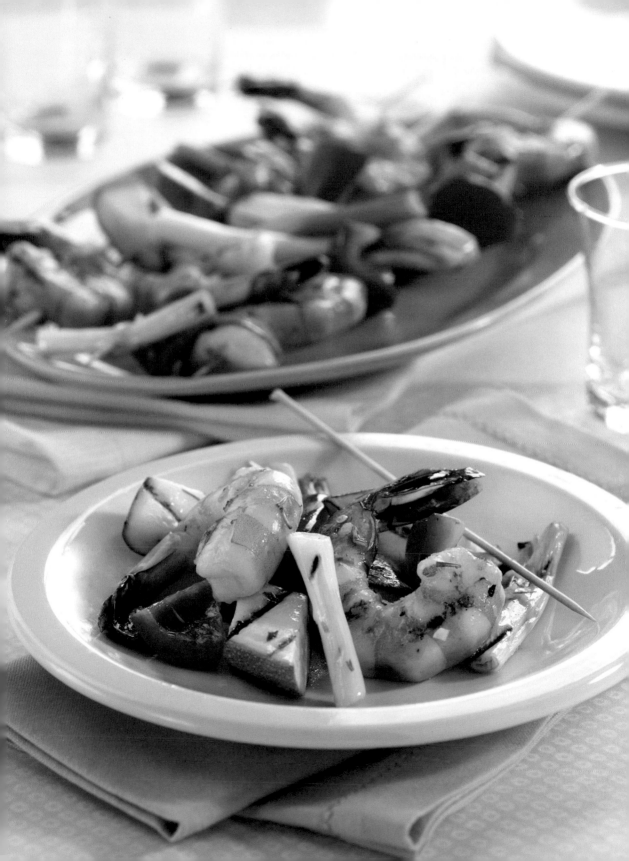

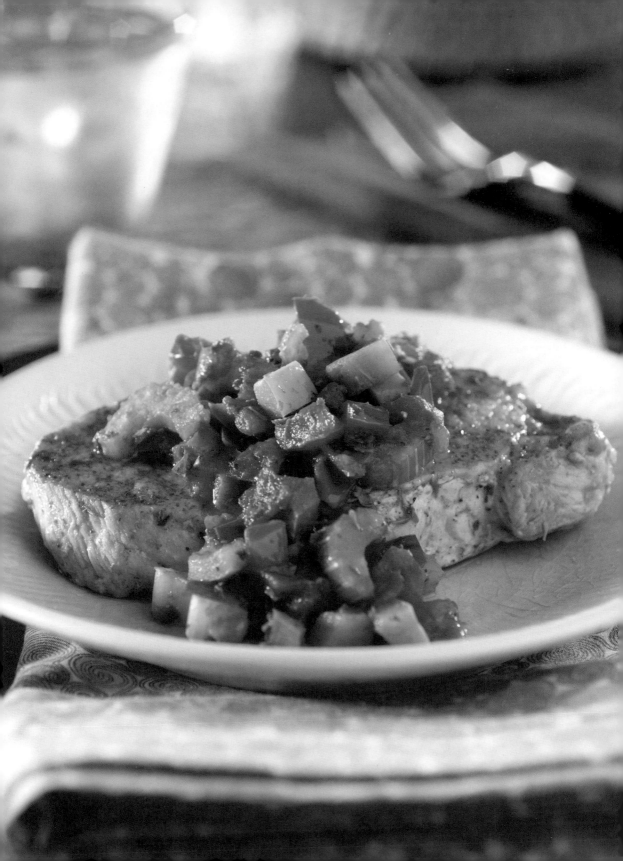

ZESTY SKILLET PORK CHOPS

1 teaspoon chili powder

½ teaspoon salt, divided

4 boneless pork chops
   (about 6 ounces each)

2 cups diced tomatoes

1 cup chopped green, red or
   yellow bell pepper

¾ cup thinly sliced celery

½ cup chopped onion

1 teaspoon dried thyme

1 tablespoon hot pepper sauce

1 tablespoon olive oil

2 tablespoons finely chopped
   fresh parsley

1. Rub chili powder and ¼ teaspoon salt over one side of pork chops.

2. Combine tomatoes, bell pepper, celery, onion, thyme and hot pepper sauce in medium bowl; mix well.

3. Heat oil in large nonstick skillet over medium-high heat. Add pork, seasoned side down; cook 1 minute. Turn pork; top with tomato mixture and bring to a boil. Reduce heat to low; cover and cook 25 minutes or until pork is tender and tomato mixture has thickened.

4. Remove pork to serving plates. Bring tomato mixture to a boil over high heat; cook 2 minutes or until most of liquid has evaporated. Remove from heat; stir in parsley and remaining ¼ teaspoon salt. Spoon sauce over pork.

MAKES 4 SERVINGS

GRILLED HALIBUT WITH CHERRY TOMATO RELISH

3 tablespoons lemon juice, divided

2 teaspoons grated lemon peel, divided

2 cloves garlic, minced

2 teaspoons olive oil, divided

½ teaspoon salt, divided

¼ teaspoon black pepper, divided

4 halibut fillets (about 6 ounces each)

2 cups cherry tomatoes, quartered

2 tablespoons chopped fresh parsley

1. Combine 2 tablespoons lemon juice, 1 teaspoon lemon peel, garlic, 1 teaspoon oil, ¼ teaspoon salt and ⅛ teaspoon pepper in large resealable food storage bag. Add halibut; seal bag and turn to coat. Marinate in refrigerator 1 hour.

2. Combine tomatoes, parsley, remaining 1 tablespoon lemon juice, 1 teaspoon lemon peel, 1 teaspoon oil, ¼ teaspoon salt and ⅛ teaspoon pepper in medium bowl; toss to coat.

3. Prepare grill for direct cooking. Spray grill rack with nonstick cooking spray. Remove fish from marinade; discard marinade.

4. Grill fish 3 to 5 minutes per side or until fish begins to flake when tested with fork. Serve with relish.

MAKES 4 SERVINGS

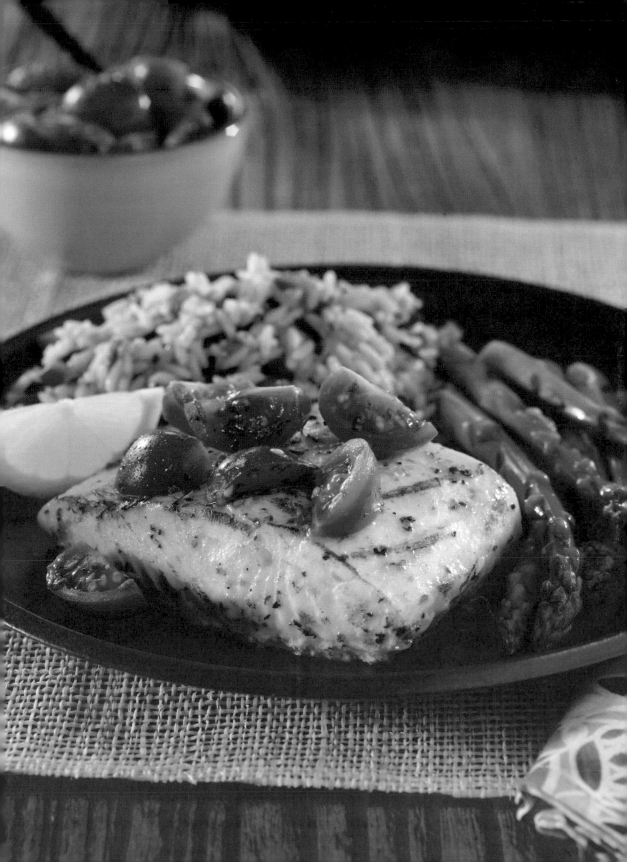

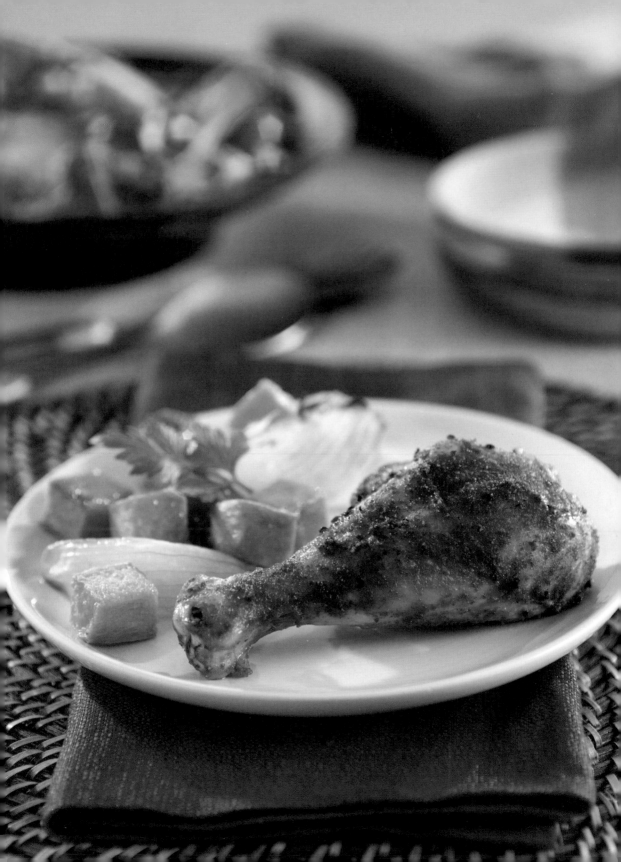

SMOKED PAPRIKA DRUMSTICKS WITH SWEET POTATOES

2 teaspoons paprika

1 teaspoon garlic powder

1 teaspoon ground cumin

¾ teaspoon black pepper

½ teaspoon salt

4 (4-ounce) or 8 (2-ounce) chicken drumsticks, skin removed

12 ounces sweet potatoes, peeled and cut into 1-inch pieces

1 medium onion, cut into 8 wedges

1 tablespoon olive oil

1. Preheat oven to 350°F. Line baking sheet with foil; spray foil with nonstick cooking spray.

2. Combine paprika, garlic powder, cumin, pepper and salt in small bowl; mix well. Coat chicken with spice mixture; place on prepared baking sheet.

3. Combine sweet potatoes, onion and oil in medium bowl; toss to coat. Arrange vegetables around chicken pieces, being careful not to crowd.

4. Roast 30 minutes. Stir vegetables and turn chicken; roast 20 minutes or until chicken is cooked through (165°F).

MAKES 4 SERVINGS

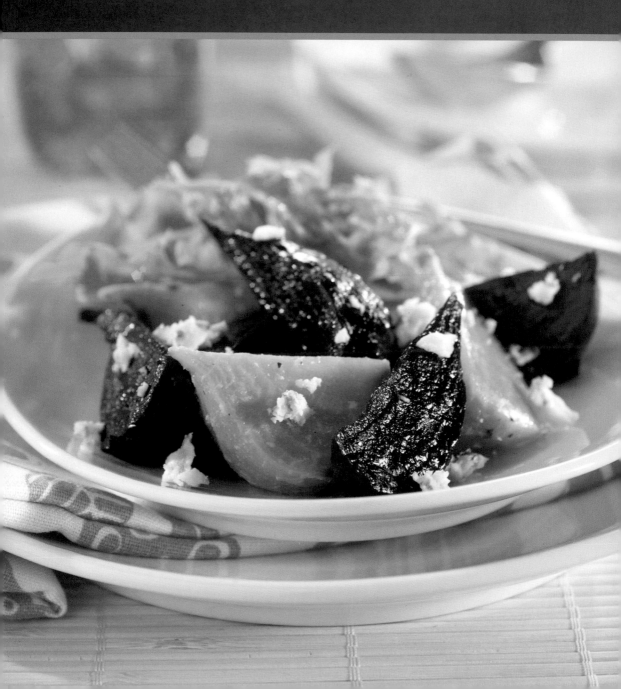

SIDE DISHES

CIDER VINAIGRETTE-GLAZED BEETS

6 medium beets

1½ tablespoons olive oil

1½ tablespoons cider vinegar

½ teaspoon prepared
   horseradish

½ teaspoon Dijon mustard

¼ teaspoon packed brown sugar

⅓ cup crumbled blue cheese
   (optional)

1. Cut tops off beets, leaving at least 1 inch of stems. Scrub beets under cold running water with soft vegetable brush, being careful not to break skins.

2. Place beets in large saucepan; add water to cover. Bring to a boil over high heat. Reduce heat to low; simmer 30 minutes or just until beets are barely firm when pierced with fork. Remove to plate to cool slightly.

3. Meanwhile, whisk oil, vinegar, horseradish, mustard and brown sugar in medium bowl until well blended.

4. When beets are cool enough to handle, peel off skins and trim off root end. Cut beets into halves, then into wedges. Add warm beets to vinaigrette; gently toss to coat. Sprinkle with cheese, if desired. Serve warm or at room temperature.

MAKES 8 SERVINGS

ROASTED POTATOES AND PEARL ONIONS

3 pounds red potatoes, scrubbed and cut into 1½-inch pieces

1 package (10 ounces) pearl onions, peeled

2 tablespoons olive oil

2 teaspoons dried basil or thyme

1 teaspoon paprika

¾ teaspoon salt

¾ teaspoon dried rosemary

¾ teaspoon black pepper

1. Preheat oven to 400°F. Spray large shallow roasting pan* with nonstick cooking spray.

2. Combine potatoes and onions in prepared pan. Drizzle with oil; toss to coat. Combine basil, paprika, salt, rosemary and pepper in small bowl; mix well. Sprinkle over potatoes and onions; toss to coat.

3. Roast 20 minutes. Stir vegetables; roast 15 to 20 minutes or until potatoes are browned and tender when pierced with fork.

Do not use glass baking dish or potatoes will not brown.

MAKES 8 SERVINGS

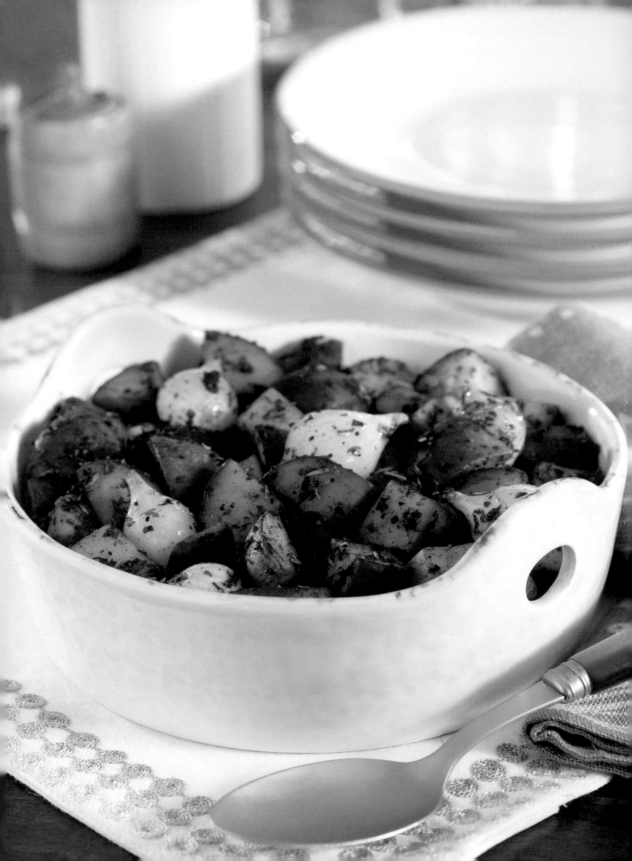

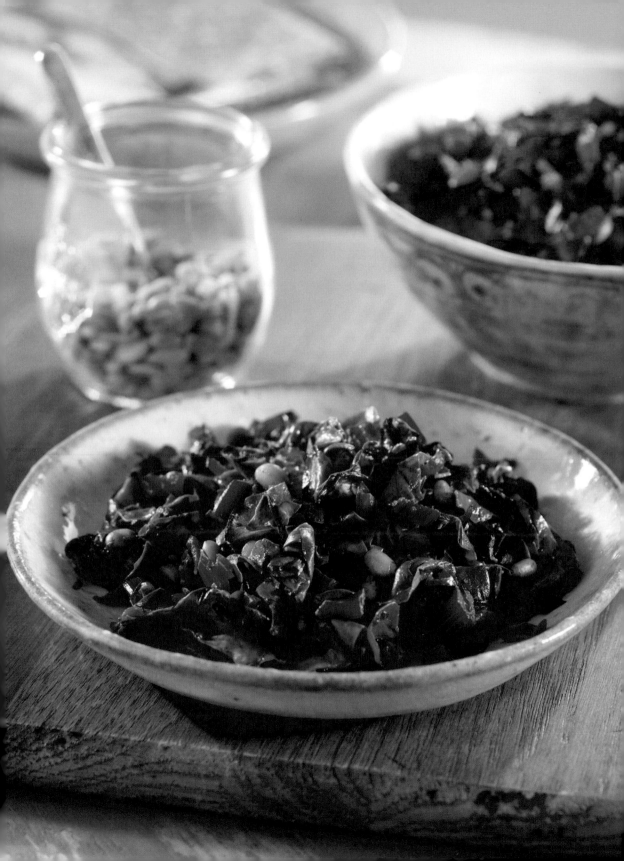

SAUTÉED SWISS CHARD

1 large bunch Swiss chard or
   kale (about 1 pound)
1 tablespoon olive oil
3 cloves garlic, minced
¾ teaspoon salt
¼ teaspoon black pepper

1 tablespoon balsamic vinegar
   (optional)
¼ cup pine nuts, toasted*

*To toast pine nuts, cook in small skillet over medium heat 1 to 2 minutes or until nuts are lightly browned, stirring frequently.

1. Rinse chard in cold water; shake off excess water but do not dry. Finely chop stems and coarsely chop leaves.

2. Heat oil in large saucepan over medium heat. Add garlic; cook and stir 2 minutes. Add chard, salt and pepper; cover and cook 2 minutes or until chard begins to wilt. Uncover; cook and stir about 5 minutes or until chard is completely wilted.

3. Stir in vinegar, if desired. Sprinkle with pine nuts just before serving.

MAKES 4 SERVINGS

SUMMER SQUASH SKILLET

2 tablespoons butter

1 medium sweet or yellow onion, thinly sliced and separated into rings

2 medium yellow squash or zucchini or 1 of each, sliced

¾ teaspoon salt

¼ teaspoon black pepper

1 large tomato, chopped

¼ cup chopped fresh basil

2 tablespoons grated Parmesan cheese

1. Melt butter in large skillet over medium-high heat. Add onion; stir to coat with butter. Cover and cook 3 minutes. Uncover; cook and stir over medium heat about 3 minutes or until onion is golden brown.

2. Add squash, salt and pepper to skillet; cover and cook 5 minutes, stirring once. Add tomato; cook, uncovered, about 2 minutes or until squash is tender. Stir in basil; sprinkle with cheese.

MAKES 4 SERVINGS

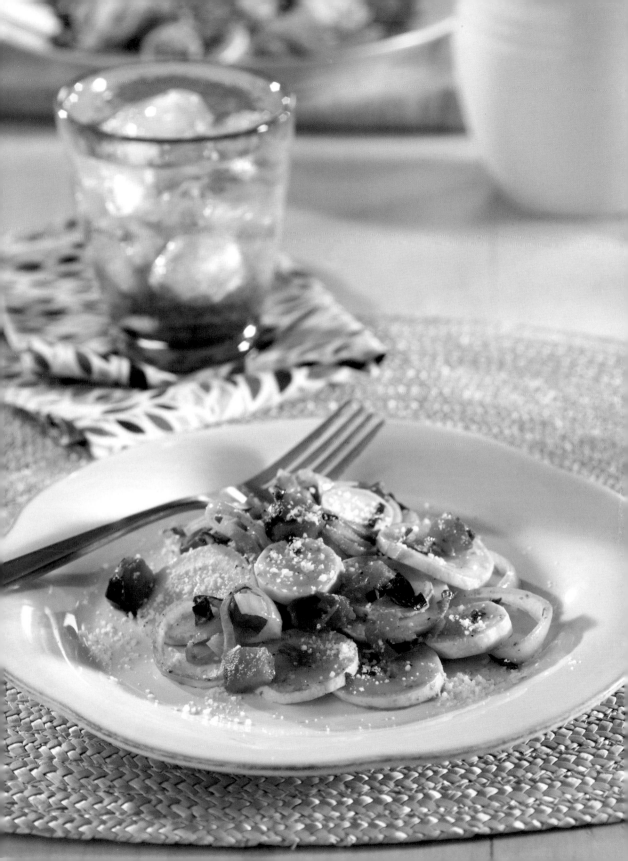

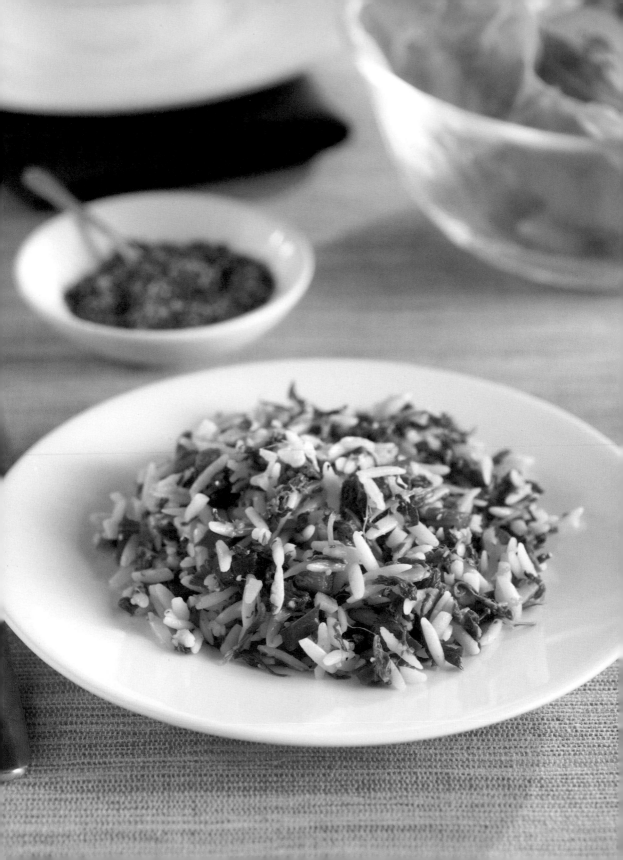

ORZO WITH SPINACH AND RED PEPPER

4 ounces uncooked orzo pasta

1 teaspoon olive oil

1 medium red bell pepper, diced

3 cloves garlic, minced

1 package (10 ounces) frozen chopped spinach, thawed and squeezed dry

¼ cup grated Parmesan cheese

½ teaspoon finely chopped fresh oregano or basil (optional)

¼ teaspoon lemon-pepper seasoning

1. Prepare orzo according to package directions; drain well.

2. Heat oil in large nonstick skillet over medium-high heat. Add bell pepper and garlic; cook and stir 2 to 3 minutes or until bell pepper is crisp-tender. Add orzo and spinach; cook and stir until heated through.

3. Stir in cheese, oregano, if desired, and lemon-pepper seasoning. Serve immediately.

MAKES 4 SERVINGS

SWEET POTATO FRIES

1 large sweet potato
  (about 8 ounces)

2 teaspoons olive oil

¼ teaspoon coarse salt

¼ teaspoon black pepper

¼ teaspoon ground red pepper

Honey or maple syrup
  (optional)

1. Preheat oven to 425°F. Lightly spray baking sheet with nonstick cooking spray.

2. Peel sweet potato; cut lengthwise into long spears. Toss with oil, salt, black pepper and ground red pepper on prepared baking sheet. Arrange sweet potato spears in single layer not touching.

3. Bake 20 to 30 minutes or until lightly browned, turning halfway through baking time. Serve with honey, if desired.

MAKES 2 SERVINGS

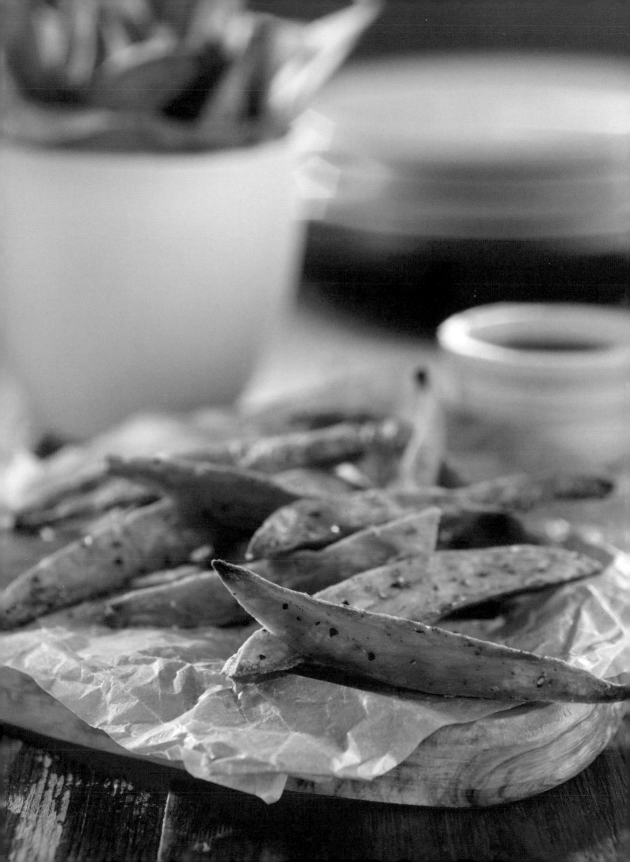

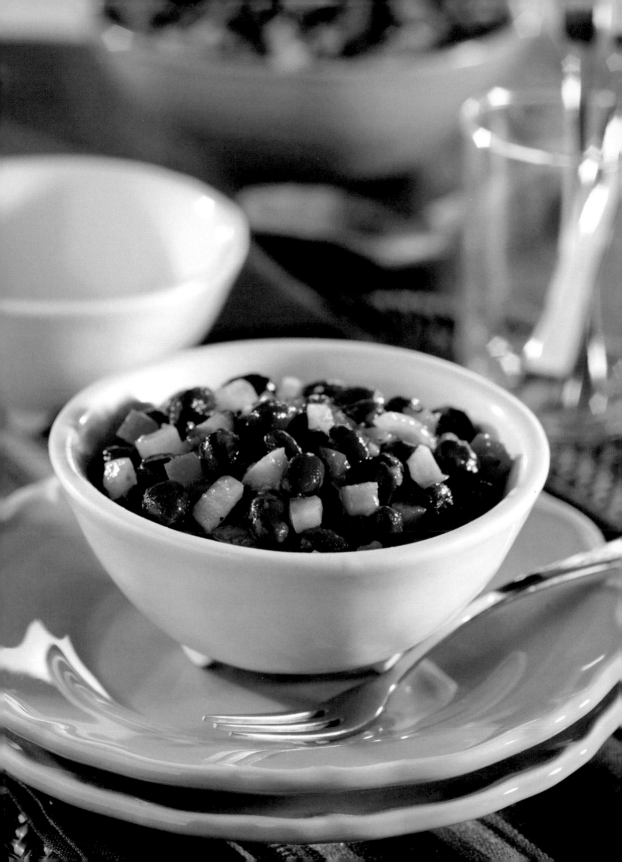

CONFETTI BLACK BEANS

1 cup dried black beans, rinsed and sorted

3 cups water

1 can (about 14 ounces) reduced-sodium chicken broth

1 bay leaf

1 tablespoon olive oil

1 medium onion, chopped

¼ cup chopped red bell pepper

¼ cup chopped yellow bell pepper

2 cloves garlic, minced

1 jalapeño pepper,* finely chopped

1 large tomato, seeded and chopped

½ teaspoon salt

⅛ teaspoon black pepper

Hot pepper sauce (optional)

*Jalapeño peppers can sting and irritate the skin, so wear rubber gloves when handling peppers and do not touch your eyes.

1. Place beans in large bowl; add water. Soak 8 hours or overnight.

2. Drain beans. Combine beans and broth in large saucepan; bring to a boil over high heat. Add bay leaf. Reduce heat to low; cover and simmer 1½ hours or until beans are tender.

3. Heat oil in large nonstick skillet over medium heat. Add onion, bell peppers, garlic and jalapeño pepper; cook and stir 8 to 10 minutes or until onion is translucent. Add tomato, salt and black pepper; cook 5 minutes.

4. Add onion mixture to beans; cook 15 to 20 minutes. Remove and discard bay leaf. Serve with hot pepper sauce, if desired.

MAKES 6 SERVINGS

ROAST ASPARAGUS WITH SHALLOT VINAIGRETTE

1 pound fresh asparagus, trimmed

4 tablespoons olive oil, divided

½ teaspoon salt, divided

1 shallot, minced

1 tablespoon balsamic or white wine vinegar

¼ teaspoon black pepper

1. Preheat oven to 425°F. Place asparagus in shallow baking pan or jelly-roll pan. Drizzle with 1 tablespoon oil and sprinkle with ¼ teaspoon salt; toss to coat.

2. Roast asparagus 10 minutes or until tender and lightly browned.

3. Meanwhile, whisk remaining 3 tablespoons oil, ¼ teaspoon salt, shallot, vinegar and pepper in small bowl until well blended. Let stand at least 5 minutes to allow flavors to blend. Spoon dressing over asparagus.

MAKES 4 SERVINGS

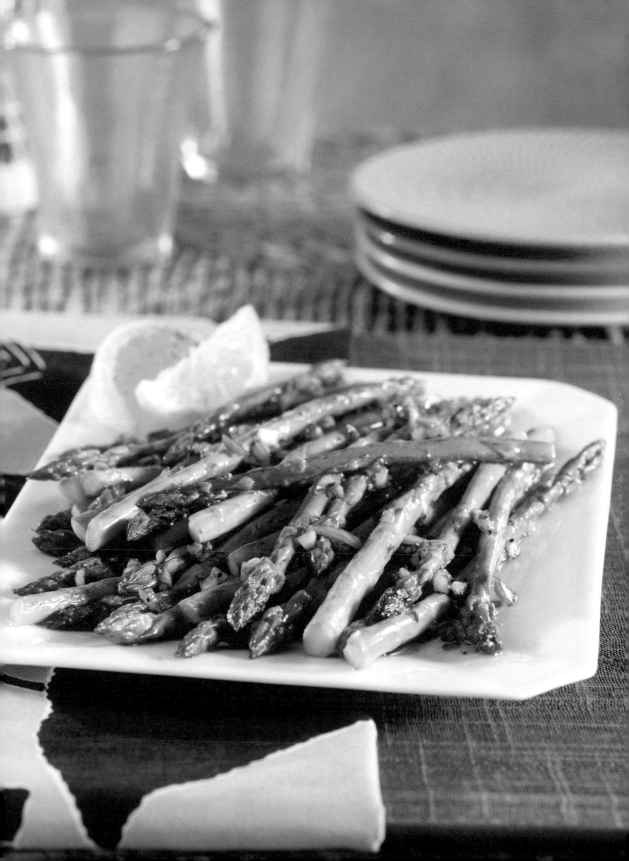

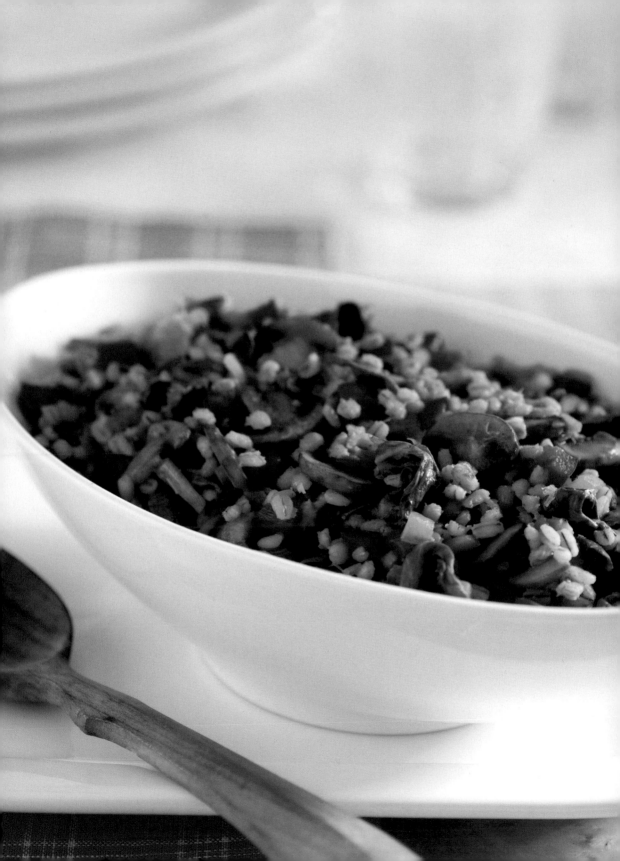

BARLEY AND VEGETABLE RISOTTO

4½ cups reduced-sodium
    vegetable or chicken broth

1 tablespoon olive oil

1 small onion, diced

8 ounces sliced mushrooms

¾ cup uncooked pearl barley

1 large red bell pepper, diced

2 cups packed baby spinach

¼ cup grated Parmesan cheese

¼ teaspoon black pepper

1. Bring broth to a boil in medium saucepan over high heat. Reduce heat to low to keep broth hot.

2. Meanwhile, heat oil in large saucepan over medium heat. Add onion; cook and stir 4 minutes. Add mushrooms; cook over medium-high heat 5 minutes or until mushrooms begin to brown and liquid evaporates, stirring frequently.

3. Add barley; cook 1 minute. Add hot broth, ¼ cup at a time, stirring constantly until broth is almost absorbed before adding the next ¼ cup. After 20 minutes of cooking, stir in bell pepper. Continue adding broth, ¼ cup at a time, until barley is tender (about 30 minutes total).

4. Stir in spinach; cook and stir 1 minute or just until spinach is wilted. Stir in cheese and black pepper.

MAKES 6 SERVINGS

Tip: Use your favorite mushrooms, such as button, crimini or shiitake, or a combination of two or more different types.

BALSAMIC BUTTERNUT SQUASH

3 tablespoons olive oil

2 tablespoons thinly sliced fresh sage (about 6 large leaves), divided

1 medium butternut squash, peeled and cut into 1-inch pieces (4 to 5 cups)

½ red onion, halved and cut into ¼-inch slices

1 teaspoon salt, divided

2½ tablespoons balsamic vinegar

¼ teaspoon black pepper

1. Heat oil in large cast iron skillet over medium-high heat. Add 1 tablespoon sage; cook and stir 3 minutes.

2. Add butternut squash, onion and ½ teaspoon salt; cook 6 minutes, stirring occasionally. (Squash should fit into crowded single layer in skillet.) Reduce heat to medium; cook 15 minutes without stirring.

3. Add vinegar, remaining ½ teaspoon salt and pepper; cook 10 minutes or until squash is tender, stirring occasionally. Stir in remaining 1 tablespoon sage; cook 1 minute.

MAKES 4 SERVINGS

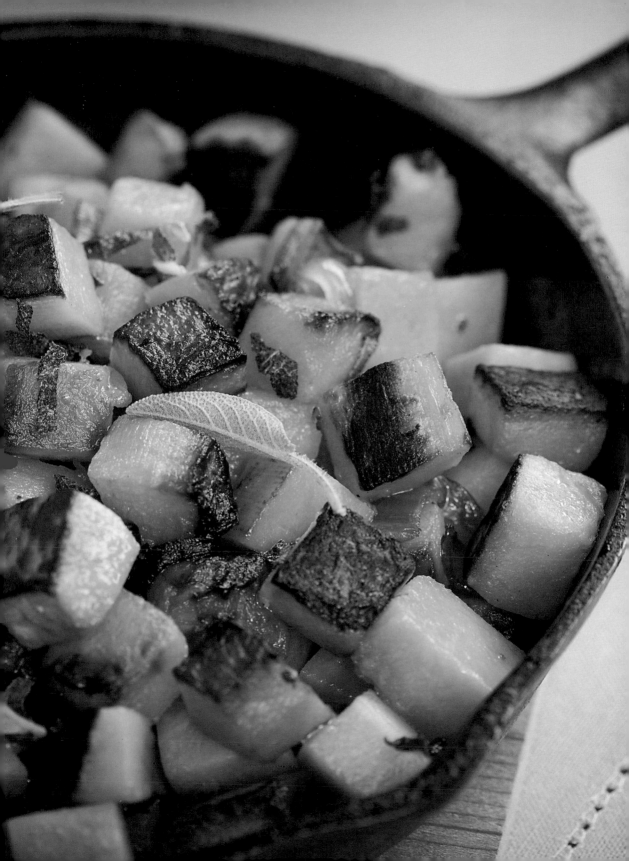

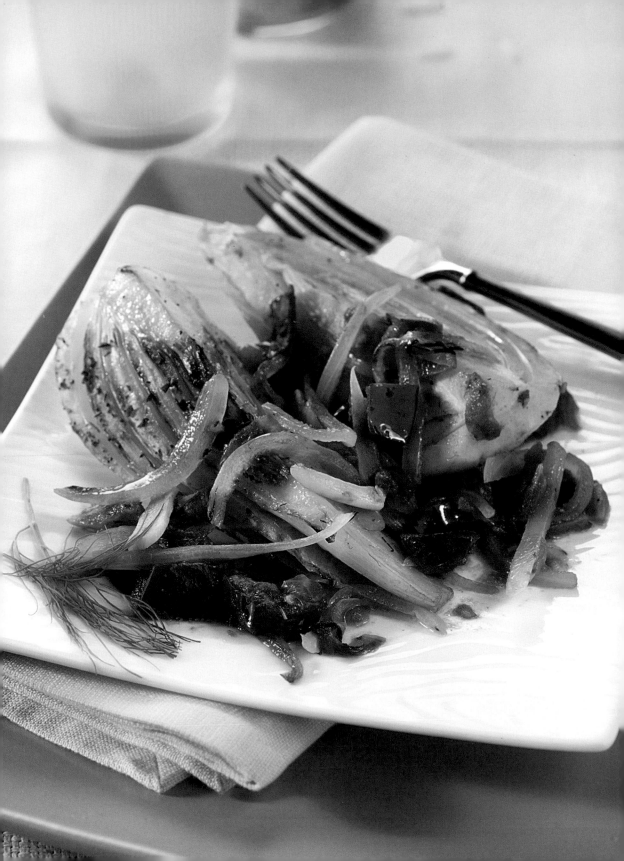

FENNEL BRAISED WITH TOMATO

2 bulbs fennel

1 tablespoon olive oil

1 small onion, sliced

1 clove garlic, sliced

4 medium tomatoes, chopped

⅔ cup reduced-sodium vegetable broth or water

3 tablespoons dry white wine or vegetable broth

1 tablespoon chopped fresh marjoram *or* 1 teaspoon dried marjoram

½ teaspoon salt

¼ teaspoon black pepper

1. Trim stems and bottoms from fennel bulbs, reserving green leafy tops for garnish. Cut each bulb lengthwise into 4 wedges.

2. Heat oil in large skillet over medium heat. Add fennel, onion and garlic; cook about 5 minutes or until onion is soft and translucent, stirring occasionally.

3. Stir in tomatoes, broth, wine, marjoram, salt and pepper. Reduce heat to low; cover and cook about 20 minutes or until fennel is tender. Garnish with reserved fennel leaves.

MAKES 6 SERVINGS

BROWN RICE WITH CRANBERRIES AND WALNUTS

1 can (about **14 ounces**) reduced-sodium vegetable or chicken broth

¾ cup uncooked brown rice or brown basmati rice

¼ cup water

½ teaspoon salt

¼ cup dried cranberries

⅛ teaspoon ground cinnamon

¼ cup coarsely chopped walnuts, toasted*

*To toast walnuts, cook in small skillet over medium heat 1 to 2 minutes or until lightly browned, stirring frequently.

1. Combine broth, rice, water and salt in large saucepan; bring to a boil over high heat. Reduce heat to low; cover and simmer 20 minutes.

2. Stir in cranberries and cinnamon; cover and simmer 20 to 25 minutes or until rice is tender. Sprinkle with walnuts just before serving.

MAKES 4 SERVINGS

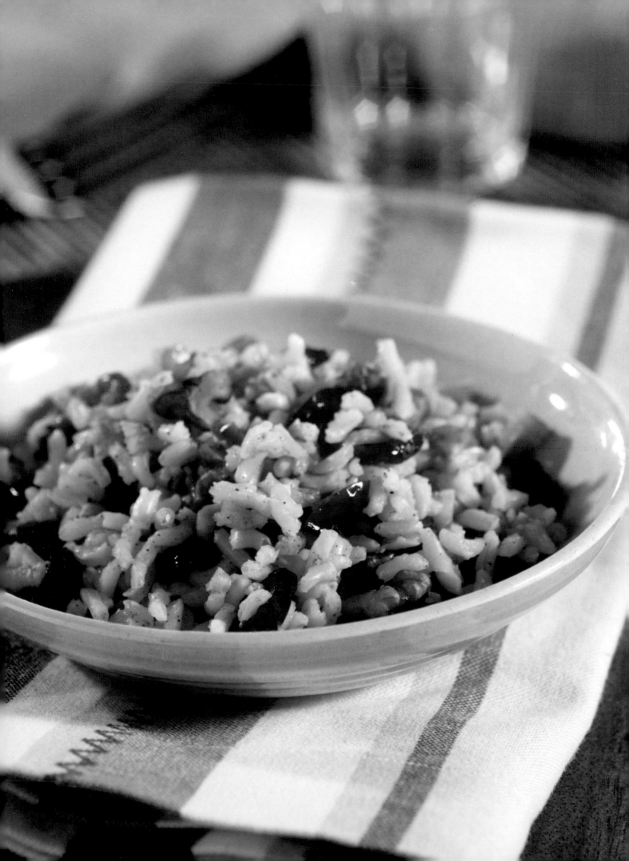

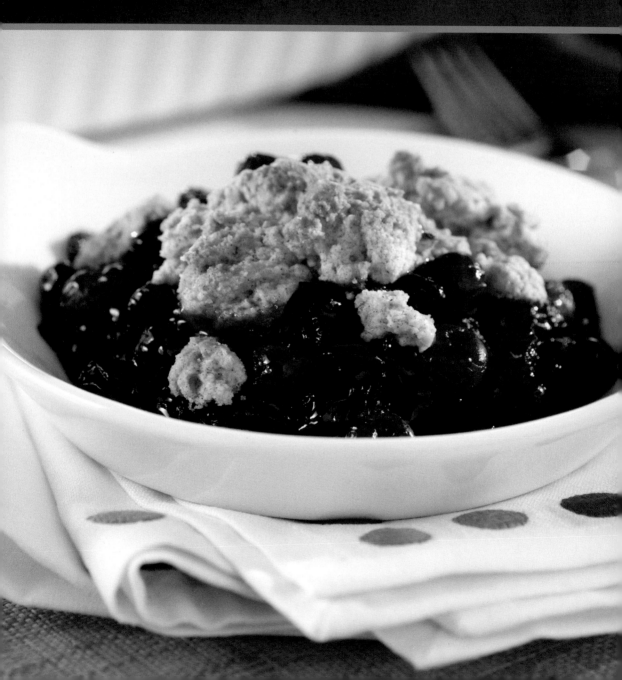

DESSERTS

TANGY CRANBERRY COBBLER

2 cups thawed frozen or fresh cranberries

1 cup dried cranberries

1 cup raisins

½ cup orange juice

¼ cup plus 2 tablespoons sugar, divided

2 teaspoons cornstarch

1 cup all-purpose flour

2 teaspoons baking powder

1 teaspoon ground cinnamon

¼ teaspoon salt

¼ cup (½ stick) cold butter, cut into small pieces

½ cup milk

1. Preheat oven to 400°F.

2. Combine cranberries, dried cranberries, raisins, orange juice, ¼ cup sugar and cornstarch in 9-inch square baking dish; toss to coat.

3. Combine flour, remaining 2 tablespoons sugar, baking powder, cinnamon and salt in large bowl; mix well. Cut in butter with pastry blender or 2 knives until mixture resembles coarse crumbs. Add milk; stir just until moistened. Drop batter by large spoonfuls over cranberry mixture.

4. Bake 35 to 40 minutes or until topping is golden brown. Serve warm.

MAKES 6 SERVINGS

BLACKBERRY SWIRL POPS

1¼ cups plain Greek yogurt

¼ cup milk

2 tablespoons sugar

2 tablespoons lime juice, divided

1 cup chopped fresh
blackberries

Pop molds

Pop sticks

1. Combine yogurt, milk, sugar and 1 tablespoon lime juice in blender or food processor; blend until smooth.

2. Combine blackberries and remaining 1 tablespoon lime juice in blender or food processor; blend until smooth.

3. Alternately layer yogurt mixture and blackberry mixture in pop molds. Using thin knife, create swirls by drawing knife up and down through layers.

4. Cover top of each mold with small piece of foil. Insert sticks through center of foil. Freeze 4 hours or until firm.

5. To remove pops from molds, remove foil and place bottoms of pops under warm running water until loosened. Press firmly on bottoms to release. (Do not twist or pull sticks.)

MAKES 6 POPS

Tip: Another way to create swirls is by using a bamboo skewer or a thin round pop stick.

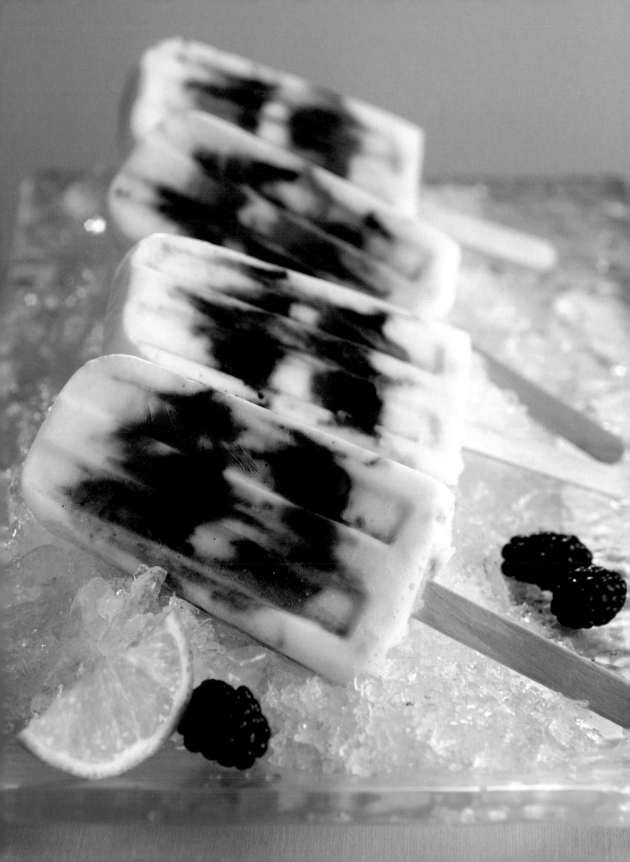

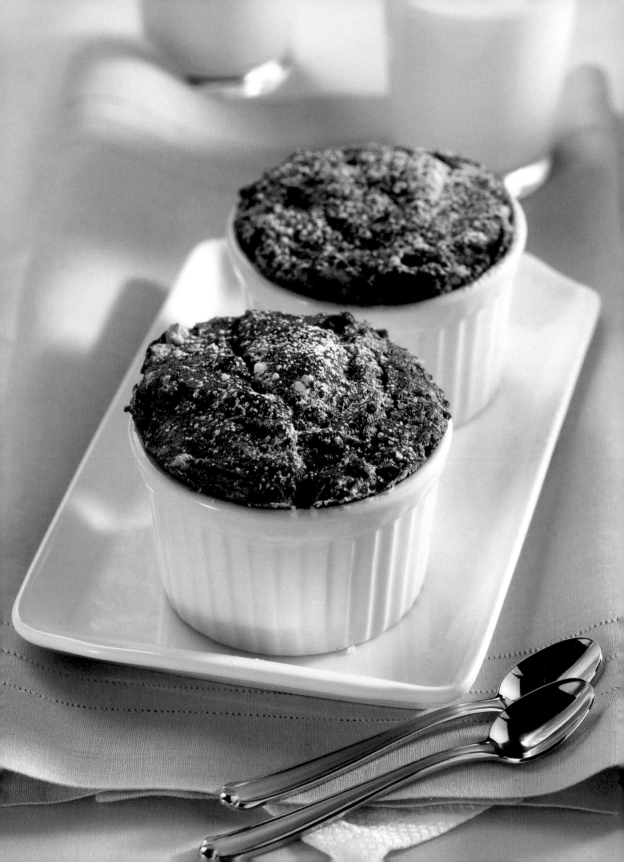

INDIVIDUAL CHOCOLATE SOUFFLÉS

1 tablespoon butter, plus additional for greasing

2 tablespoons plus 1 teaspoon sugar, divided

4 ounces bittersweet chocolate, broken into pieces

2 eggs, separated, at room temperature

Powdered sugar (optional)

1. Preheat oven to 375°F. Coat 2 (6-ounce) soufflé dishes or ramekins with butter. Add ½ teaspoon sugar to each dish; shake to coat bottoms and sides.

2. Combine chocolate and 1 tablespoon butter in top of double boiler; heat over simmering water until chocolate is melted and smooth, stirring occasionally. Remove from heat; stir in egg yolks, one at a time, until blended. (Mixture may become grainy, but will smooth out with addition of egg whites.)

3. Beat egg whites in medium bowl with electric mixer at high speed until soft peaks form. Gradually add remaining 2 tablespoons sugar; beat until stiff peaks form and mixture is glossy.

4. Gently fold egg whites into chocolate mixture. Do not overmix; allow some white streaks to remain. Divide batter evenly between prepared dishes.

5. Bake 15 minutes until soufflés rise but remain moist in centers. Sprinkle with powdered sugar, if desired. Serve immediately.

MAKES 2 SOUFFLÉS

Tip: Add a pinch of cream of tartar to the egg whites before beating to make a stronger egg white foam.

BERRY-QUINOA PARFAITS

⅔ cup uncooked quinoa

2 cups plus 2 tablespoons milk,
    divided

⅛ teaspoon salt

¼ cup sugar

1 egg

1½ teaspoons vanilla

2 cups sliced fresh strawberries

¼ cup vanilla yogurt

Ground cinnamon (optional)

1. Place quinoa in fine-mesh strainer; rinse well under cold water. Combine quinoa, 2 cups milk and salt in medium saucepan; bring to a simmer over medium heat. Reduce heat to medium-low; simmer, uncovered, 20 to 25 minutes or until quinoa is tender, stirring frequently.

2. Whisk remaining 2 tablespoons milk, sugar, egg and vanilla in medium bowl until well blended. Gradually whisk ½ cup hot quinoa mixture into egg mixture, then whisk mixture back into saucepan. Cook over medium heat 3 to 5 minutes or until bubbly and thickened, stirring constantly. Remove from heat; let cool 30 minutes.

3. Layer quinoa mixture and strawberries in 6 parfait dishes. Top with dollop of yogurt; sprinkle with cinnamon, if desired.

MAKES 6 SERVINGS

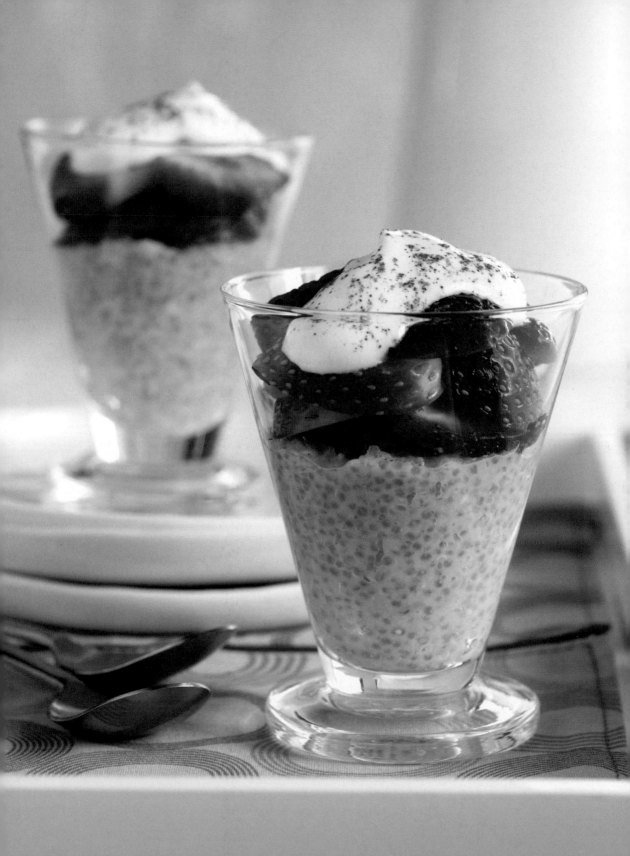

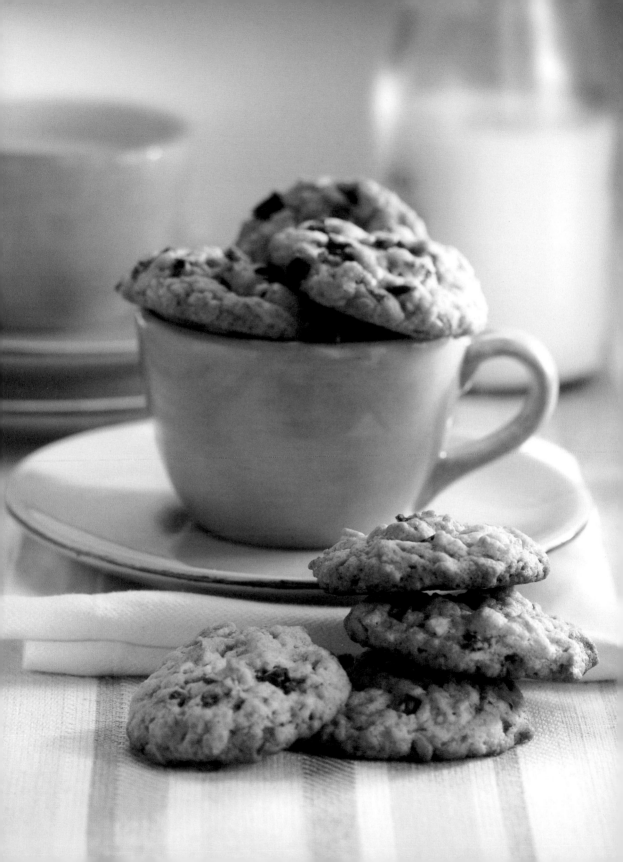

PEANUT BUTTER OAT CHIP MINI COOKIES

⅓ cup granulated sugar

⅓ cup butter, softened

¼ cup packed brown sugar

¼ cup creamy peanut butter

1 egg

½ teaspoon vanilla

1 cup quick oats

⅓ cup all-purpose flour

¼ cup whole wheat flour

½ teaspoon baking powder

¼ teaspoon baking soda

¼ teaspoon salt

⅓ cup mini semisweet chocolate chips

¼ cup dried cherries, coarsely chopped

1. Preheat oven to 375°F.

2. Beat granulated sugar, butter, brown sugar and peanut butter in large bowl with electric mixer at medium speed until creamy. Add egg and vanilla; beat until well blended. Add oats, all-purpose flour, whole wheat flour, baking powder, baking soda and salt; beat at low speed until blended. Stir in chocolate chips and cherries. Drop mixture by slightly rounded teaspoonfuls onto ungreased baking sheets.

3. Bake 8 to 9 minutes or until edges are lightly browned. Cool on cookie sheets 1 minute; remove to wire racks to cool completely.

MAKES ABOUT 50 MINI COOKIES

STRABERRIES WITH >> HONEYED YOGURT SAUCE

1 cup plain yogurt

1 tablespoon orange juice

1 to 2 teaspoons honey

⅛ teaspoon ground cinnamon

1 quart fresh strawberries, hulled

Combine yogurt, juice, honey and cinnamon in small bowl; mix well. Serve sauce over strawberries.

MAKES 4 SERVINGS

FRUIT KABOBS WITH RASPBERRY DIP

½ cup vanilla Greek yogurt

¼ cup raspberry fruit spread

1 pint fresh strawberries, hulled

2 cups cubed honeydew melon (1-inch cubes)

2 cups cubed cantaloupe (1-inch cubes)

1 can (8 ounces) pineapple chunks in juice, drained

1. Combine yogurt and fruit spread in small bowl; mix well.

2. Thread fruit alternately onto 6 (12-inch) skewers. Serve with yogurt dip.

MAKES 6 SERVINGS

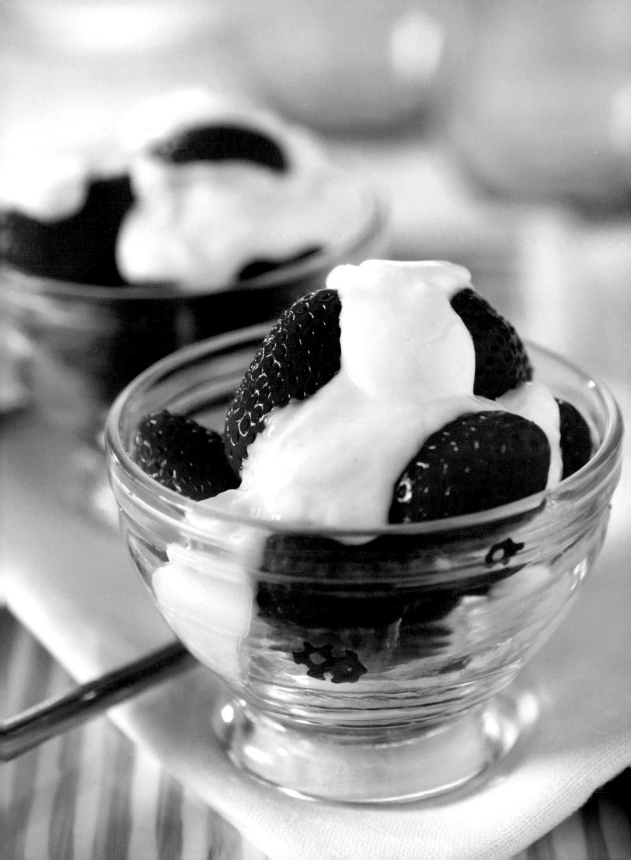

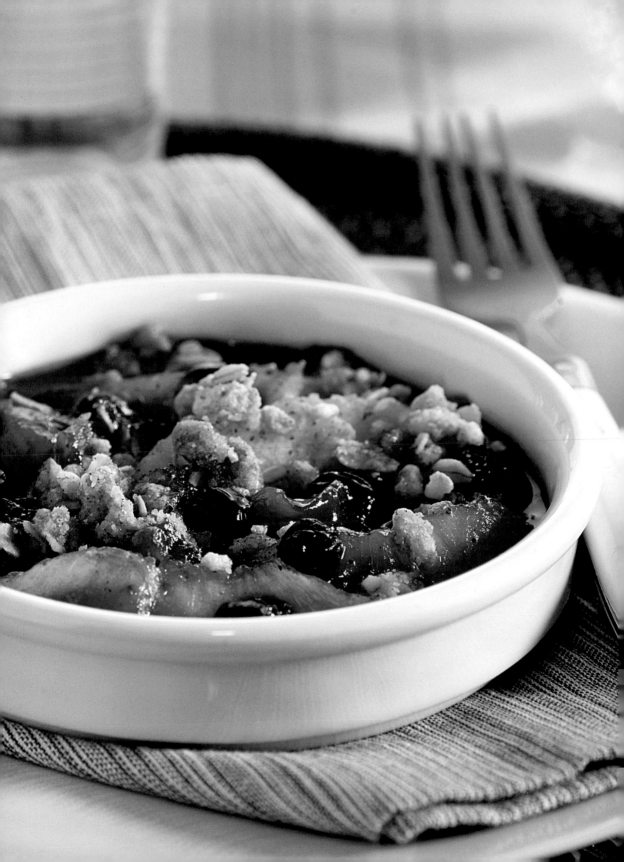

PEACH AND BLUEBERRY CRISP

3 cups fresh or thawed frozen sliced peeled peaches, undrained

1 cup fresh or thawed frozen blueberries, undrained

2 tablespoons granulated sugar

¼ teaspoon ground nutmeg

2 tablespoons old-fashioned oats

2 tablespoons crisp rice cereal

2 tablespoons all-purpose flour

1 tablespoon packed brown sugar

1 tablespoon butter, melted

⅛ teaspoon ground cinnamon

1. Preheat oven to 375°F.

2. Combine peaches and blueberries in ungreased 8-inch round cake pan. Combine granulated sugar and nutmeg in small bowl; mix well. Sprinkle over fruit; toss gently to coat.

3. Combine oats, cereal, flour, brown sugar, butter and cinnamon in small bowl; mix well. Sprinkle over fruit mixture.

4. Bake 35 to 40 minutes or until peaches are tender and topping is golden brown.

MAKES 4 SERVINGS

PINEAPPLE-LIME SORBET

1   ripe pineapple, cut into cubes
    (about 4 cups)
⅓   cup frozen limeade
    concentrate

1   to 2 tablespoons lime juice
1   teaspoon grated lime peel,
    plus addtional for garnish

1. Arrange pineapple in single layer on large baking sheet; freeze at least 1 hour or until very firm.*

2. Combine frozen pineapple, limeade concentrate, lime juice and 1 teaspoon lime peel in food processor or blender; process until smooth and fluffy. If mixture doesn't become smooth and fluffy, let stand 30 minutes to soften slightly; repeat processing. Serve immediately. Garnish with additional lime peel.

*Pineapple can be frozen up to 1 month in resealable freezer food storage bags.

MAKES 8 SERVINGS

Note: This dessert is best if served immediately, but it can be made ahead, stored in the freezer and then softened several minutes before being served.

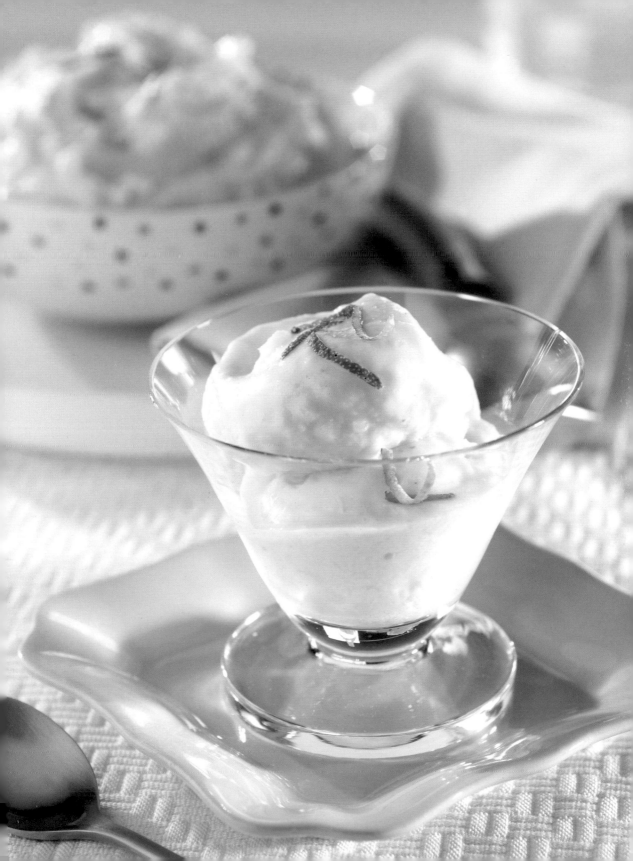

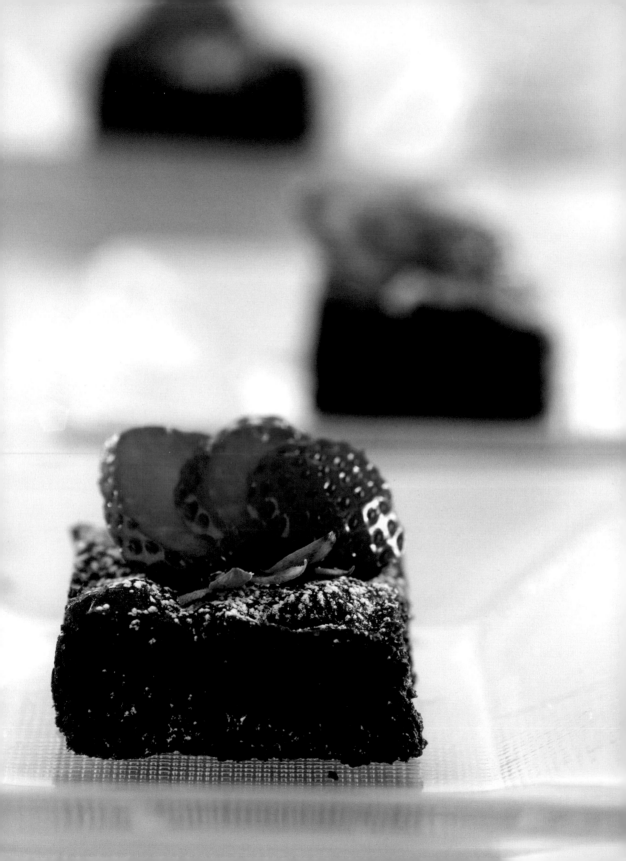

WHOLE WHEAT BROWNIES

½ cup whole wheat flour

½ teaspoon baking soda

¼ teaspoon salt

½ cup (1 stick) butter

1 cup packed brown sugar

½ cup unsweetened cocoa
   powder

2 eggs

½ cup semisweet chocolate
   chips

1 teaspoon vanilla

Fresh strawberries (optional)

1. Preheat oven to 350°F. Spray 8-inch square baking pan with nonstick cooking spray.

2. Combine flour, baking soda and salt in small bowl; mix well. Melt butter in large saucepan over low heat. Add brown sugar; cook and stir about 4 minutes or until sugar is completely dissolved and mixture is smooth. Remove pan from heat; stir in cocoa until smooth. Stir in flour mixture until blended. Beat in eggs, one at a time, until blended. Stir in chocolate chips and vanilla. Spoon batter into prepared pan.

3. Bake 15 to 20 minutes or until toothpick inserted into center comes out almost clean. Garnish with strawberries.

MAKES 16 BROWNIES

METRIC CONVERSION CHART

VOLUME MEASUREMENTS (dry)

1/8 teaspoon = 0.5 mL
1/4 teaspoon = 1 mL
1/2 teaspoon = 2 mL
3/4 teaspoon = 4 mL
1 teaspoon = 5 mL
1 tablespoon = 15 mL
2 tablespoons = 30 mL
1/4 cup = 60 mL
1/3 cup = 75 mL
1/2 cup = 125 mL
2/3 cup = 150 mL
3/4 cup = 175 mL
1 cup = 250 mL
2 cups = 1 pint = 500 mL
3 cups = 750 mL
4 cups = 1 quart = 1 L

VOLUME MEASUREMENTS (fluid)

1 fluid ounce (2 tablespoons) = 30 mL
4 fluid ounces (1/2 cup) = 125 mL
8 fluid ounces (1 cup) = 250 mL
12 fluid ounces (1 1/2 cups) = 375 mL
16 fluid ounces (2 cups) = 500 mL

WEIGHTS (mass)

1/2 ounce = 15 g
1 ounce = 30 g
3 ounces = 90 g
4 ounces = 120 g
8 ounces = 225 g
10 ounces = 285 g
12 ounces = 360 g
16 ounces = 1 pound = 450 g

DIMENSIONS

1/16 inch = 2 mm
1/8 inch = 3 mm
1/4 inch = 6 mm
1/2 inch = 1.5 cm
3/4 inch = 2 cm
1 inch = 2.5 cm

OVEN TEMPERATURES

250°F = 120°C
275°F = 140°C
300°F = 150°C
325°F = 160°C
350°F = 180°C
375°F = 190°C
400°F = 200°C
425°F = 220°C
450°F = 230°C

BAKING PAN SIZES

Utensil	Size in Inches/Quarts	Metric Volume	Size in Centimeters
Baking or Cake Pan (square or rectangular)	8×8×2	2 L	20×20×5
	9×9×2	2.5 L	23×23×5
	12×8×2	3 L	30×20×5
	13×9×2	3.5 L	33×23×5
Loaf Pan	8×4×3	1.5 L	20×10×7
	9×5×3	2 L	23×13×7
Round Layer Cake Pan	8×1½	1.2 L	20×4
	9×1½	1.5 L	23×4
Pie Plate	8×1¼	750 mL	20×3
	9×1¼	1 L	23×3
Baking Dish or Casserole	1 quart	1 L	—
	1½ quart	1.5 L	—
	2 quart	2 L	—